The Nice Guys' Guide™ To Getting Girls 2

You CAN be a Nice Guy & STILL Attract Women!

*by The Nice Guys' Institute™
featuring The Nice Guy™ (John Fate)
and The Nice Guys™*

Edited by
Betsy Ayres Smith

Please e-mail us at:
TheNiceGuys@TheNiceGuysGuide.com

ajackal publishing
Chesapeake VA

Visit our website at www.TheNiceGuysGuide.com
Contact us at TheNiceGuys@TheNiceGuysGuide.com

Visit Ajackal Publishing website at www.ajackal.com

First printing 2004

ISBN   0-9746042-9-1

LCCN   2003098286

Library of Congress Cataloging-in-Publication Data
The Nice Guys' Guide™ To Getting Girls 2: You CAN be a Nice Guy & STILL Attract Women! / The Nice Guys' Institute™ featuring The Nice Guy™ (John Fate) and The Nice Guys™.
P.cm.
ISBN: 0974604291

CONTENTS

To Oscar, the original Nice Guy

ACKNOWLEDGMENTS

Editor: *Betsy Ayres Smith*

This book also includes some content originally intended for use in The Nice Guys' Guide to Getting Girls™, previously edited by Laura Nathan.

Cover Design: *Joseph Williams*

Thanks to all of our families and friends, for all that you've taught us about relationships.

– The Nice Guy™
and The Nice Guys™

Other Products by The Nice Guys™:

Make Every Girl Want You™
by John Fate (The Nice Guy™*), Steve Reil*

The Nice Guys' Guide to Getting Girls™

The Nice Guys' Guide™ *Audio Series*

Please see www.TheNiceGuysGuide.com for
the latest from The Nice Guys' Institute™!

The Nice Guys™ have appeared on:

The O'Reilly Factor

The Other Half

MTV's Big Urban Myth Show

The Ricki Lake Show

Naked New York

Jamie (White) & Danny (Bonaduce) Show

Don & Mike

Bubba the Love Sponge

Bottom Line Radio

Elvis Duran & The Z Morning Zoo

The Morning Madhouse

FNX Morning Show

Paul & Young Ron

...and others, too numerous to name!

WARNING—DISCLAIMER

Chapter 1 – The Nice Guys' Guide™ Introduction

This book is really the third in *The Nice Guys' Guide™* Series. It is intended to be a sequel to both *The Nice Guys' Guide to Getting Girls™* and *Make Every Girl Want You™*. We wrote those books – and this one – not because we were natural-born ladies' men looking to teach some old dogs new tricks, but because we know firsthand what it's like to go for months or even years without a date. Back in college, there was a good chance that if you looked up the word "pathetic" in the dictionary, you would find the definition followed by, "See also: 'John Fate.'" In those days, John didn't just fail miserably at wooing women to sleep with him – much less date him! – but he couldn't get women to give him the time of day if his life depended on it. It often felt as if every woman on earth had signed a pact and agreed not to acknowledge his very existence.

Oh, sure, if the girl sitting next to him in class didn't understand something, she might ask him for clarification. He might have even chatted with her briefly during class. But if he saw her at a bar or a frat party later that night, he would be lucky if he got more than a thirty-second conversation out of her. Truth be told, he was usually not even that lucky.

Why was he so pathetic? And why were all of us at The Nice Guys' Institute™ originally so pathetic? Because we were all "nice guys." Maybe you can relate to this. To this very day, we are still nice guys. And that's about all we've got going for us. We're not rich, we're not famous, and we're not particularly good-looking. One of the first things we recognized, when we started observing why we were so pathetic, is that there are three categories of guys who seem to get all of the women. Guys who are:

1. Rich,
2. Famous, or
3. Good-looking

Unfortunately, like 90% of the other guys in this world, we have none of these three things going for us. We are not rich, not famous, and not good-looking; we are all merely average, nice guys.

For a period of time during college, in fact, John was so desperate for a date that he decided to abandon his natural "nice guy" personality for a while. He thought that acting like a rich, famous, or good-looking guy might cause the women to finally flock to him – or at least give him the time of day – so he put on this cocky, arrogant attitude when approaching the gender that we all desire. Since this series isn't entitled *The Jerk's Guide to Getting Girls*, you've probably guessed correctly that this plan backfired. Although John didn't think it was possible, women wanted to be around him even less when he acted like someone he wasn't! So the moral to the story is that if you're not rich, famous, or good-looking, don't try to pretend you are and expect to reap some sort of benefit. Nice guys like us need our own approach to women.

After he graduated from college, John was so fed up with his pathetic life that he, and his good friend

Steve, decided they had to take action. Thinking like the engineering majors that they were, they decided to take an analytical approach to studying women. So, they came up with a game plan: For the next few months, they would only try to befriend women. They wouldn't try to date them; they wouldn't try to sleep with them. They would simply make it a point to become friends with every woman they met.

John and Steve began implementing this plan, and within a few months, they had a few dozen female friends! They would go out to bars and parties with these women and observe other guys hitting on them. They learned what worked and what didn't. The best part was that since they were friends with these women, these women would debrief John and Steve after guys hit on them. The women would say things like:

> "Ugh, I can't believe that guy wouldn't shut up about med school."

> "Wow, that guy had the most beautiful eyes!"

> "Ugh, did that guy seriously think I wanted to hear non-stop about his boat? Talk about self-absorbed!"

> "Wow, I really enjoyed talking to that guy. I didn't even feel like he was hitting on me."

While constantly capitalizing on the expertise of their newfound female friends, John and Steve also began studying their friend Oscar. Oscar, the nicest guy you'll ever meet, was a completely average guy like all of us: not rich, not famous, and not exceptionally good-looking. Yet, somehow, Oscar was constantly surrounded by beautiful women. Oscar was always dating these women; he was always sleeping with these women. Oscar had a date whenever he wanted one. His success with women was an enigma to all of us, so we decided that we would study Oscar to figure out what it was about this seemingly-average nice guy that made him so attractive to women.

Make Every Girl Want You™ was John's and Steve's first attempt to share everything they learned about women with guys. Because of the tremendous success of that book, John then started The Nice Guys' Institute™, which seeks to help other "nice guys" make themselves more desirable to women without turning into jerks. And John recruited us, The Nice Guys™, to assist in that mission.

In the pages that follow, we have attempted to answer the most common questions that we've received from you, the readers of *Make Every Girl Want You*™ and *The Nice Guys' Guide to Getting Girls*™, and the attendees of our courses. First, a word of warning: Much of the material in this book is written with the assumption that you have read *Make Every Girl Want You*™ and *The Nice Guys' Guide to Getting Girls*™. Many of the concepts as well as the terminology introduced in those books provide the basis for this follow-up book; therefore, we strongly advise you to at least peruse the previous books before reading any further.

Written in a stream of consciousness style, this book is comprised of a series of articles that address specific questions posed to us, in the courses we've taught, through the thousands of e-mails we've received, in the hundreds of interviews we've conducted, or things that have naturally occurred to us as we experience life. As with *Make Every Girl Want You*™ and *The Nice Guys' Guide to Getting Girls*™, the advice in this book is based on everything we've learned from our observation of and conversations with two sources:

1. Our many female friends
2. Oscar

Oscar epitomizes what every guy wants to be – a truly nice guy whom women love. Nowadays, as the founder of The Nice Guys' Institute™, John is frequently referred to as The Nice Guy™. However, John always says that Oscar was the original Nice Guy since none of us can imagine that there would've been a Nice Guys' Institute™ if Oscar hadn't inspired John.

Before we move on to the substance of the book, let us briefly answer a question that we hear every time one of us teaches a course:

> "Why don't you just ask Oscar how he does it?!?"

We've tried that, but unfortunately, it's not really something that he can explain. Oscar has never taken the time to ponder why so many women are attracted to him. He just behaves the way that was naturally engrained in him, which we're sure was some magical combination of genetics and his upbringing, such that everything in him somehow aligned to create the perfect Nice Guy. If only we could all be so lucky. Since Oscar didn't even have the answer to our million-dollar question, all we could do was watch, observe, and take notes. Hopefully, you'll like what we've learned. So read on to find out how to be a Nice Guy and *still* be attractive to women!

But first, we'd like to close this chapter the way we have with our previous books, by presenting six of our favorite testimonials. Since the release of the first books in *The Nice Guys' Guide*™ Series, we have received thousands of testimonials, both from men and women, thanking us for our books and courses. We'd now like to present six of our favorites, to illustrate how our books and courses have helped others, and how they will help you too.

From Robert, a 34-year-old man who has been married for eight years:

"Our marriage had reached the point where we'd only had sex 3 times in the last 5 years. I wasn't even sure if she still loved me anymore.

I tried a million things, bringing her flowers, taking her out to nice dinners, buying her jewelry. Still nothing. I couldn't even get her to talk about what was wrong with our marriage. Then, a friend of mine got me your book on a whim. He said, 'Hey, Robert. Try reading this. It might help.' And it did, this has changed my life!

Not only is our sex life improved, but I feel like, for the first time in about 5 or 6 years, my wife and I actually understand each other. And we enjoy spending time together once again. Thanks...for saving my marriage."

From Michael, a 19-year-old college student:

"I've never had much luck with girls. In fact, as much as it hurts me to write this, I made it to 19 as a virgin. Don't get me wrong, I've been out on dates. But I guess the problem is that I can never get to the 3rd date, if you know what I mean. I just really had no clue how to behave on a date. I read your book cover to cover, and then went back and read it a 2nd time.

A week later, I was sitting next to this really hot girl in my chemistry class. I struck up a conversation, exactly as you guys instructed. That weekend, I found myself having sushi with her. Only this date was different. It was unlike any date I've ever been on. I could tell that she was actually digging me! I don't think she looked at her watch once the entire time.

Best thing is, I didn't even need a 3rd date, because 3 nights later we went out again and she had sex with me! Thank you. Thank you. Thank you."

From Lisa, a single gal who withheld her age:

"I bought a copy for my friend, Harold. Harold's a great guy. I've been friends with him for 8 years, and let me just say that he has not had much success with the ladies. Which really isn't fair, because he's the world's sweetest guy. Of course, as a woman, I can kind of understand why he doesn't have success with women. But the thing is, as much as I've tried to explain it to him, he just doesn't get it.

So I heard you guys on a radio show, and decided to buy your book for him. You guys said in 150 pages what I haven't been able to get Harold to understand in 8 years! Harold just has so much more confidence now. I can tell when I'm around him that he actually, finally, feels comfortable interacting with women. Sure, he's not a walking, talking babe magnet, but he's so much better off.

In fact, I recently introduced him to a couple of my female friends, who have both since asked about him. I mean, *my* friends – asking about Harold? That just doesn't happen! I'm almost starting to get jealous! Thanks guys, for a great book. I think every girl should buy it for her platonic male friends!"

From Corey, a 25-year-old professional:

> "It's been a few years since I graduated from college. I have a good job and live in the city now, but man it's so much tougher to meet women than it was in college. In college, there were girls over at the frat house all the time. It was so easy to hook-up. Now, I can't even figure out where to meet women, let alone hook-up.
>
> I ordered your book, and read it cover to cover in an hour. I discovered that my main problem is that I was looking for girls in all of the wrong places. Great book, guys—thanks a ton. I've already told all of my friends about it."

From Roger, who is 37 years old and divorced:

> "I finally understand why my first marriage failed. And let me tell you, until now I was clueless. I read your guys' book, because I'm single now. And I really read it for tips on where to meet women. But what really helped me is that you pointed out every single thing I did wrong in my first marriage.
>
> I'm dating someone now, and I definitely want to get married again someday. I don't know if it'll be to her, but I feel like I finally know what it will take to make a marriage work. I would recommend your book to any guy who wants to make his second marriage work."

From Julia, who is married—happily now—and requested that we not print her age:

"I've been trying for years to get Bill to read 'relationship books.' But I haven't been able to get him to read a damn one. I saw you guys on TV, and figured—what the hell—I'll get your book, basically as a last resort. I gave it to Bill, and he read the entire thing that night.

Afterward, he came up to me, gave me a big hug, and said: 'Honey, I have 2 things to tell you. #1: I want you to know how beautiful you are. And #2: I'm sorry I haven't told you that in 13 years.'"

Part I The Nice Guys' Guide™ to Meeting Women

In the "Meeting Women" section of The Nice Guys' Guide to Getting Girls™, we offered advice on where to meet women, and how to approach women in different types of environments, such as airports, gyms, and cruises. We also talked about criteria to use when evaluating whether or not you're in the right bar to meet women. Finally, we authored the official guide to meeting women online. In Part I of The Nice Guys' Guide 2™, we will offer further advice on where to meet women, from meeting women online to meeting women through female friends, that we at The Nice Guys' Institute™ have discovered since our last book.

Chapter 2 – The Nice Guys' Guide™ to More Online Dating

In *The Nice Guys' Guide to Getting Girls*™, we started the official guide to online dating. We advised you how to fill out your profile, write your initial e-mail, post your photo, and meet the woman for the first time. We touched upon out-of-town online dating, and we even included some sample e-mail exchanges between a friend of ours and a woman he met through Match.com. Yet, we still get tons of e-mails from guys, asking us to preview their "standard online response e-mail," to tell them what they're doing wrong. It is impossible for us to provide feedback to everyone, so we included this chapter in the book.

We at The Nice Guys' Institute™, being the research mavens that we are, decided to conduct a little experiment. We wanted to see what it would be like to be a beautiful woman, and how guys would respond to her. So we created a fake profile, using a picture of a model from a clothing catalog, and posted her profile on Match.com. We made her 22 years old, with a fake address in the heart of New York City. Here is the profile we created, and posted online for her:

> Headline: Sweet girl
>
> I'm a funny, caring, and loving girl. I love to make people laugh and be there for them when they need someone. I love the ocean and anything that has to do with it. I was a dancer for 11 years and a cheerleader for 4 years and I still remain extremely athletic. I work out almost everyday of the week. Alright, can't reveal too much... you can find the rest out later...
>
> I'm looking for someone who is understanding, honest, funny, and compassionate. Of course, good looks are a +, but I need an intelligent man that can treat me right and always be there for me.

We posted the ad at night and then went to bed. By noon the following morning, we had already received fifty responses from guys in the New York area, all vying for her (our) attention! During the first week after we posted that picture, we received an average of forty to fifty e-mails a day from guys!

Next we decided to ask four of our female friends, Amanda, Jessica, Mia, and Beth, all of who have participated in online dating, to analyze the dozens of responses we had received from guys, as if the response was sent to them. These are the most enlightening responses. Hopefully you will find some things in these e-mails that you have been doing, and see how our female friends reacted to them, so you can apply this critique to your own e-mails.

One final note: all e-mails appear "as is." We did not correct spelling or grammatical errors, so you could see for yourself exactly how guys respond online.

> **Case Study**: "What's up? My name is [deleted]. I'm a very mature 22 year-old from Nassau county. I work in the city full time and enjoy pretty much anything. I enjoy going to bars and clubs and dancing my azz off. If your interested in more and want some pixs, e-mail me at [e-mail address deleted]. Or if you have IM, you can IM me at the same address.
>
> P.S. You have very beautiful eyes. I bet you hear that all the time. ;)"

> Amanda: "Dancing his azz off, huh?"

> Jessica: "Yeah, although that's kind of cute. What really bothers me here is that he doesn't show the least bit of interest in me. Totally looks like something he fired off to a dozen women."

> Mia: "Yeah, he's very mature but enjoys dancing his azz off. At least he has a job though. And he made an attempt to compliment me."

> **Case Study**: "I have never tried the internet dating scene before but will try anything once. I must say your Ad left me pleasantly surprised and intrigued!
>
> I am a young professional looking for a good time and hopefully someone special. I am 6'2" 185 pounds with a muscular

build. My sign is Leo and I have blue eyes with brown hair. Some people say I look like Mathew Perry and others say Leonardo Dicaprio. I think they just look like me ;), although not as plump as Mathew and not as skinny as Leo.

I am very active, my hobbies are (in no particular order) snowboarding, mountain biking, going to the gym, museums, travel, dining out, Broadway shows, movies, photography, coffee houses, people watching and of course sports. As active as I am I don't mind staying in and catching a flick from time to time. I am finishing up grad school but work part time as a real estate broker. I have never been married and don't smoke but I do drink occasionally. My three main goals in life are too be happy, successful, and healthy. Five things I can't live without are good food, good times, good friends, family, and TRAVEL! I am pretty open minded so if you are looking for a prince give me a shout!"

Mia: "He seems very honest from the beginning. I like the way he humorously compared himself to celebrities. Leo and Matthew – good mix! Definitely seems to have his life together, and comes across as a pretty sincere, down-to-earth guy. I'd definitely consider e-mailing him back."

Jessica: "Yeah, the one thing that bothers me is no interest shown in me! I'm definitely big on that. Anything that looks like he fired it off to a few dozen women and that guy's out."

Case Study: "My names [name deleted]. I think I fit your understanding, honest, compassionate, and intelligent qualifications, but as for funny, well I think you'll have to find that out for youself:P We seem to have working out in common as for anything else im not sure because you havent said much. So take a look at my profile and if your interested I'd liek to hear more about you."

Beth: "OK. Criticizing me from the beginning... not a way to win me over! Don't tell me that I haven't said much... I know that already! And nice ability to repeat, verbatim, back the things I told you I'm looking for in a guy."

Jessica: "Well, at least he took the time to read my profile. Didn't really say much to intrigue me though."

Amanda: "Apparently this guy's too lazy to use apostrophes or spell-check."

Case Study: "Hello there, My name is [name deleted] and I wanted to respond. I liked the way you described yourself and thought your pictures were very attractive. I am 35, 5'11", and have blonde hair and blue eyes. I have recently returned to NY (from San Francisco), work in fiance, and like the company of smart, interesting people that are fun to be around and who appreciate an unconventional sense of humor.

I'm attaching a picture of myself. Please let me know if you're interested and we can chat some more.

Best wishes,
[name deleted]
[e-mail address deleted]

PS: It blocked my picture when I sent it, so hopefully I will be able to resend it upon your reply."

Beth: "OK, none of this 'can't send my picture stuff.' If I took the time to scan in my picture, and post it on Match.com for the world to see, then you had better take 5 minutes to do the same. The fact that this guy a) won't post his picture in public, and b) is making excuses for why he can't send it through e-mail, is a big turn-off. No response back from me."

Mia: "He works in fiancé??? I don't even want to know what that means!"

Jessica: "I think he meant finance, but yeah – not taking the time to re-read his e-mail... bad form.

Amanda: "Unconventional sense of humor? What does that mean? I'm a little scared."

Beth: "Yeah, does that mean he's gonna sit there and fart all during dinner? Or is he gonna tell me a bunch of offensive jokes? I'm scared too!"

Case Study: "we should try to talk

i can send you my picture if you want
send me and e-mail
[e-mail address deleted]
talk with you soon"

Beth: "And I thought that last guy was scary!"

Amanda: "Um, no."

Jessica: "Delete!"

Mia: "Next!"

Case Study: "Hey Alyssa,

Such a fitting name :) ... Well, I really like your profile, especially the part about oceans and staying athletic! I would really like to get to know you better too, so if you'd like to chat more write me back.

I'm attaching a picture of myself with a friend of mine. (I'm the one on the left in the white shirt.)

Greg"

Amanda: "Such a fitting name??? What the hell does that mean?!?!"

Jessica: "Give him a little credit, he did take the time to at least peruse my profile."

Mia: "Why do guys always do that??? I'm attaching a picture of me and all of my frat brothers in front of the fraternity house. I'm the sixth one from the left, in between Biffo and Bongo, smoking a cigar."

Beth: "Can we e-mail him back and ask if his friend's single?"

Amanda: "Yeah, his friend's *way* hotter!"

Case Study: "I guess i'll start by saying that i didn't name myself oceanboy for nothing. I'm all about the ocean, and like you say anything that has to do with it.

I am 25 years old. I am 5'10', brown hair and eyes, sort of olivish skin too. (i will immediately send you a photo if you would like) I live in jersy. 20 minutes west of the city. I am going to be a second year law student in the fall, and for the summer i am working for a judge in lower manhattan.

bottom line. I pride myself in moderation....I like to party with the best of them, but also love just chilling out with friends whenever the moment is right.

I spend the weekends during the summer at the beach. I like to go out one night in the city and then cruise down at some strange hour.

I am very energetic. I rowed at georgetown, and continue keeping fit by running everyday and playing tennis when i have chance.

what else....I can't think of much now, but I assure you there's plenty more, so i hope this interests you, and like i said, i would definitely love to send you a photo if you would like.

best

ocean boy."

Beth: "No photo. No dice."

Jessica: "I like how he tried to connect with me through the ocean. Pretty cool that his screen name was ocean boy, especially since we said in our profile that we love the ocean."

Mia: "Yeah, ocean boy is cute and all, but what's your real name??? You forgot to mention it!"

Beth: "You know, it's sad. Most of what this guy has to say is actually pretty attractive. Loves to have fun. Lives life in moderation. But he still makes a few key errors. No photo, and no name mentioned. That gives me the creeps. Is he really a 25-year-old law student, or a 45-year-old married guy?"

Case Study: "Hi! I loved your profile! You seem very feminine. I especially like it that you described yourself as funny and caring.

I'm a 28-year-old attorney. I'm 5'11" 170 with short dark hair and green eyes. I like dancing, musicals, concerts, operas. I'm also a big fan of travel, most recently having returned from Portugal.

Tell me more about yourself. Have you been to the ocean recently? What is your idea of a good date?

Hope to hear from you soon,

[name deleted]"

Mia: "I seem very feminine? Thank you. You seem very masculine. What does that mean, by the way?"

Beth: "Yeah, I don't know about this guy. I don't want to read into things too much, but he seems like a very traditional guy. You know, he wants to be the lawyer, the head of the household. While I sit at home and take care of the kids. And we're meeting an awful lot of lawyers, aren't we? Are there really this many lawyers in New York City?"

Jessica: "Not bad. Had some interesting things to say. But what about ME? You know, the girl on the other end of the e-mail?? ME? How about showing some interest in me? Anybody? If I ever do this online thing again for real, and a single guy actually shows interest in me, I'm his for life!"

Case Study: "Hi, I saw your profile and was very interested in writing. The silly match thing says we are a good match, who knows, but I think your smile is great? A little about me I guess would be a good start, my name is [name deleted] and I just turned 36, I am 6'2", 205lbs, blonde hair, green eyes and in good shape. I live in NJ and work in Midtown as a Systems Director for an investment bank. I love to do tons, I love the city, going to shows, dinners, museums, art galleries, walking around and just enjoying everything it has to offer. In the past few summers I spend a lot of time down the shore either at friends or I have had my own share in several houses. I like to travel, enjoy going to islands, Vegas, AC or just anyplace is great with the right person. I think I am generally a very happy person, I like my job and I think that is very important as that sort of sets the tone for the day. I am looking to find someone who has a similar outlook on life and is interested in sharing it all with someone special. I guess that's a bunch to start with for now. Let me know if you would be interested? I didn't post a pic on here as I am a little skeptical, but do have a few I could send if you are still interested?

I look forward in hearing from you,

[name deleted]"

Jessica: "He sure had a lot to say. Especially for someone who didn't even read my profile!!"

Amanda: "He was kind of sweet. Definitely had some cool things to say. No pic, no response though."

Now that you have seen how four of our friends responded to these e-mails, hopefully you know what *not* to do if you decide to meet women online. We'll now spend the rest of this chapter addressing some of your most commonly asked questions.

QUESTION: You guys say, when it comes to online dating, to take the time and read through a woman's profile. In your initial e-mail to her, you should mention some things she talked about in her profile. The problem is I have to fire off so many e-mails before I'll even get one woman to respond that I just don't have the time to send them each an individual e-mail. I don't have the time to read through each woman's profile and send her a personalized e-mail. How do you handle this?

ANSWER: You're right, that is a major conundrum for guys in the online dating world. As we stated in *The Nice Guys' Guide*™, the odds of any one woman responding to your initial e-mail are very slim, so in order to ensure that you get a few responses, it is a necessity that you fire off e-mails to a few dozen women. This then creates the conundrum: how can you e-mail so many women, and take the time to write them each an individualized e-mail?

What we have found works the best is to have a standard template that you e-mail to everyone. In there, you should change one, two, or maybe three lines, depending on what the woman says in her profile. That way you only need to take a few seconds reading through a woman's profile to pick out some things to pop into your template, but at least you convey to the woman that you did take the time to read her profile and learn something about her.

As you can see by the responses from our female friends earlier in this chapter, it is key that you take the time to personalize at least a few lines in your response back to her. Otherwise she'll think it's a template that you fired off to every other woman, and women really don't like that.

QUESTION: I met this girl online and we seemed to really hit it off. We e-mailed back and forth for hours at a time and finally met in person. When we met in person, we were both a little nervous but we really seemed to hit it off. It appeared that we both had a great time. She even stressed that she was really excited to go out with me again after that.

Then when I got home that night after our date, I logged back on to match.com to see if any other women had e-mailed me back. When I logged on, I noticed that she, too, was now online checking for messages. Does this mean the date didn't go as well as I thought it did, if she's looking for responses from other guys? Am I being a hypocrite because I did the same thing? And finally, do you think that she saw I was logged on and is now wondering the same thing?

ANSWER: Whoa, this brings up a good point that we here at The Nice Guys' Institute™ never really thought about before – going out on a date with someone and then coming home and having her see you log back on to match.com. In fact, this problem isn't merely confined to a date. You may have been exchanging some great e-mails with a woman, when she notices that you also spent the next eight hours online. We're pretty sure this doesn't send too positive of an impression to a woman either.

Is there a solution? Some online dating websites have a built-in blocker that lets you hide your name from certain people when you're online. In some cases, it's person-specific. You can specifically block one or two women from seeing that you're online. If this is the case, utilize it. After you've gone on a date with a woman, block her so she can never again see that you're back on that web site. If there's a woman who you've been e-mailing back and forth with, you should probably also block her from being able to see that you're online, so that she doesn't suspect that you're spending hours online chatting with other women (because, while there's nothing wrong with dating or chatting with other women online, it still sends a negative impression to other women). We asked our friend Emily how she would handle this situation:

> "Hmmm... that's something I really hadn't thought about. But yeah, if I'd just gone out with a guy, and came home and saw him checking out other women online, I'd be really turned-off and disappointed. I guess it's hypocritical of me though, because the only way I'd know if he was logged-on is if I was logged-on myself.
>
> But, I don't know, if I've just gotten back from a great date with someone, it kind of kills the whole romance of it to see him online, probably chatting with other women. I guess the moral of the story – for guys and women – is to all block our screen names once we've started dating someone, so they don't catch us online chatting with other people!"

The answer to your question is probably not to worry about it too much. She probably didn't notice that you were online. If the two of you had a great time together, then it shouldn't really matter anyway. Thank you very much, though, for making this excellent point to us, and allowing us to share your findings and provide a solution for other guys.

QUESTION: I live in a big city, but I live way outside of the city in a pretty remote suburb. I created an online account and started searching and responding to women who live within five miles of me. I chose five miles because traffic in the city is awful and I really don't want to travel too far to meet a woman. There seemed to be plenty of available women, even within only five miles of me.

Now here's my dilemma. Apparently I ended up e-mailing two girls who were friends with each other. One of them never responded back to me but I'd actually been exchanging e-mails with the other one and things seemed to be going pretty well... until I found out that the two girls knew each other. The one whom I had been e-mailing confronted me about this by e-mail. She actually forwarded me the similar e-mail that I had sent to her friend with a mean note at the top saying, "Hey, I thought you really meant these things you say. Apparently you're e-mailing this to every girl in the city."

Where did I go wrong? I followed your advice. I sent a templated e-mail, only changing a few things in every e-mail, and sent it out to a few dozen women. I'm glad I did that because I only got three responses. Had I not sent it out to that many women, I wouldn't have gotten any responses. How can I avoid this in the future?

ANSWER: This is another big problem you've uncovered in the world of online dating. It seems like the best thing to do is to expand your search area. You may not want to drive more than a few minutes to meet a woman, but to avoid this happening in the future, it's probably best to search for women who live within 20-30 miles of you. This should ensure that you're reaching a diverse group of women who probably don't know each other. Unfortunately, however, it seems like every once in a while, this problem would occur, especially since a lot of the women we know joined these online sites together, almost as a dare from one to the other.

From our experience, you will frequently end up e-mailing women who are friends with each other. That's why it is extremely important to search for women across a large distance, such as the 20 or 30 miles that we recommended, and not simply confining your search to within five miles of your home. One of our friends, Anna, had this pertinent advice to share about her online dating experience:

> "Yeah, I joined an online dating site but only because a couple of my friends were doing it too, and we agreed that we would do it together. Overall it's been a lot of fun. None of us has met a great guy, but it's still fun to get dozens of e-mails a day from random guys. As for your question about any of us getting e-mails from the same guy, I'm sure it happens all the time but to be honest, we all get so many e-mails every day that I'm sure we'd have no way of knowing even if we got the same exact e-mail from the same exact guy.

> But yes, we do compare e-mails from each other. For example, if we get a really bad one, I'll forward it on to my girlfriends or if they get a really good one, they'll forward it on to me and ask if they should respond. But overall, most of the e-mails that I get remain unread in my inbox because I just get too many to read all of them. So even if I got an e-mail from my girlfriends of a guy they were really intrigued by, odds are I may have gotten the same e-mail but just never got around to opening it. I guess that's just the breaks in online dating, in this new world of dating."

QUESTION: How many times is too many to e-mail a girl? I mean, let's be honest, most of the women I e-mail never get back to me. Can I keep e-mailing them repeatedly hoping they'll get back to me?

ANSWER: You probably shouldn't e-mail a woman more than two times. The first time a woman doesn't respond you can assume that it's because she was so inundated with e-mails from guys that she never got around to reading yours. The second time she doesn't respond, you should probably cease e-mailing her further, and assume that she isn't interested in you. You certainly don't want to keep e-mailing a woman to the point that she thinks you're a stalker and calls the police on you.

As we have previously discussed, you never know when one of these girls who isn't e-mailing you back is best friends with another girl that you've also been e-mailing. In that case, consider yourself lucky that one of the women never e-mailed you back, before they realize that you've been e-mailing them both! It is probably best after two e-mails to refrain from e-mailing an unresponsive woman any more.

QUESTION: After exchanging a few e-mails with a woman, I searched the internet on her, and found out quite a lot of things about her. In one of our e-mail exchanges, I brought up something that she hadn't yet told me about. I had just found it on some web page. She immediately became irate, accused me of cyber-stalking her, and cut off all future contact with me. What went wrong?

ANSWER: Never reveal to a woman anything that you've learned about her that she hasn't already told you on her own. This applies to both the online and offline worlds of dating. It's usually very easy to figure out quite a bit of information about someone by using the Internet. For example, if she gives you her full name, you can often find a woman's phone number, address, and e-mail address. Hell, you can sometimes access her credit report. You can also enter the woman's name into search engines and learn a lot about her. For instance, you can often find out where a woman went to school and what hobbies she participated in, simply by searching websites that have her name.

To reiterate very bluntly: do *not* share any information that you have learned about a woman by "cyber stalking" her. We have actually seen guys who are so proud of their cyber stalking abilities that they e-mail women with the information they learned about the women. For whatever reason, these guys think that women are impressed by their savvy Internet expertise. Cyber stalking has exactly the opposite effect – it scares the living hell out of these women! Our friend Rachel relates what happened to her:

> "Oh, my God! This guy e-mailed me back and he knew so much information about me. He knew where I'd gone to school. He knew that I played on the school soccer team. He knew what sorority I was in. He had my personal e-mail address. He had my alumni e-mail address. It was scary. The tone he related it to me, it was like he was proud that he had all this information on me.
>
> Now I'm sure the guy was completely harmless and meant nothing by it but it scared the living hell out of me. This random guy is stalking me in cyberspace because I gave him my name and phone number. I've definitely learned a lesson from this. From now on, I'm staying completely anonymous until I've met the guy in public a couple of times and I know that I trust him."

QUESTION: Hey, I love The Nice Guys' books. You guys are the greatest. I have a question for you, though. You guys are big promoters of e-mailing as many women as possible on online dating sites, to increase your odds that one will respond. Well, when a few respond and you find yourself e-mailing them all, how in the world do you keep track of what you've told to whom??

ANSWER: Always keep notes of your correspondence with women online. Most of the time, when you pursue Internet dating, it's difficult to initially get the ball rolling. You often have to send out a few dozen e-mails before you even get one response. Over time, however, you'll start corresponding with a few women. It's crucial to jot down some notes any time a girl shares anything with you, or any time you share something with her. The easiest thing to do is to keep a pad and a pen right by your computer. As you e-mail a girl, quickly jot down a couple of things that you told her and as she e-mails you back, jot down a couple of things you've learned about her. If you keep your notes about each girl on a different page of the pad, then you'll be able to keep what you've learned about each girl separate from the others.

Before you meet a girl in person for the first time review your notes about her, to remind yourself of everything that you've learned about her, and what you've already shared with her about yourself. Nothing is more embarrassing than e-mailing a girl for two weeks, meeting her in person, and not remembering which girl she is or a single thing that she has told you over the last two weeks. Our good friend Autumn related this experience:

> "I met this guy on the Internet and we spent a week and a half shooting e-mails back and forth to each other. Oh, I shared so much with him. He seemed like the perfect guy. Everything was going so well,

so we finally met in person. One of the first things he asked me about was how my cat was doing. Well, I don't have a cat. He then proceeded to bring up where I went to school, which was wrong, and he even mistakenly thought I'd been married before. It became pretty obvious after a while that he'd been e-mailing other women online and obviously couldn't remember which one I was.

After a while we got to laughing about it. He apologized profusely and we actually did have a great time together, but I really couldn't let myself see him again after that mistake. It's a shame too because I felt like we probably could have had something. The chemistry was there and everything, but I just couldn't accept the fact that he'd been e-mailing a bunch of other women and couldn't even take the time to review my e-mails before meeting me to remember which one I was.

Honestly, I wasn't bothered so much by the fact that he was e-mailing other women, because hey, I too was e-mailing other guys. What bothered me the most was that, before we went out, I took the time to read back through all of his e-mails, so everything he'd shared with me was fresh on my mind. He couldn't even take a few minutes before meeting me in person to review my e-mails and that really bothered me, it really put me off."

As you can see, there is no excuse for forgetting what a woman has shared with you over e-mail.

A final option is, if you're too lazy to even write notes onto a pad, to write all of your e-mails in word processing software (such as Microsoft Word) and saving them. Additionally, when you get responses back from a woman, copy the text out of her e-mail message and paste it into Microsoft Word, and then save that file with her name. If you save your files with names such as: "To Autumn 1", "To Autumn 2", "To Autumn 3", "From Autumn 1", "From Autumn 2", "From Autumn 3", you will have a directory of files that you can read through before meeting a woman in person, to remind yourself of everything the two of you have shared with each other.

There's nothing wrong with saving women's e-mails and reviewing them before you meet in person. As our friend Autumn shared, women do it too. It's much better than the opposite – confusing her with another woman that you've been e-mailing!

As the online dating craze is rapidly evolving, we at The Nice Guys' Institute™ are constantly doing more research, and running more experiments, to keep you informed. Please visit www.TheNiceGuysGuide.com to learn about our latest findings.

Visit the site often as we are constantly updating it with new content, including downloadable e-books and e-reports, audio tapes and CDs, and video cassettes and DVDs packed with our latest discoveries. We also maintain information on our web site about upcoming coaching sessions, course offerings, and speaking engagements. Additionally, we encourage readers to e-mail us, either through our web site, or at TheNiceGuys@TheNiceGuysGuide.com. Finally, please also come by and sign up for our free newsletter to receive the hottest tips to help nice guys like you make themselves more attractive to women WITHOUT turning into jerks!

Chapter 3 – The Nice Guys' Guide™ to Friendships with Women

In previous books in *The Nice Guys' Guide*™ Series, we have talked about the tremendous value of having friendships with women. We discussed how female friendships provide the best outlet for meeting other women (in fact, this is how we are introduced to most of the women we meet). Additionally, we discussed the concept of vouching and the three types of incredible vouches that your female friends can provide (Direct, Indirect, and Subconscious).

When you walk into a party with a beautiful platonic female friend by your side, every other woman in the room will take notice. Even if they find out that the two of you are just friends, women will be just as impressed that you're able to have a platonic friendship with a beautiful female without having it turn into something sexual.

We've found that some of the best women to have as female friends are women with boyfriends or husbands. This is especially true if her boyfriend or husband works long hours, is in med school or law school, lives out of town, or is stationed overseas. Women in these situations are often looking for new friends and for new ways to spend their time since their boyfriends or husbands are often not around. We've found that these women love it when we befriend them and invite them to do fun things with us and our friends, such as going out on a friend's boat, going to a backyard cookout, or going to a football game.

A quick disclaimer before we continue: This chapter is *not* meant to encourage infidelity. We are not suggesting that you go out and meet women with boyfriends and husbands so they can cheat on their boyfriend or husband with you. Not at all. We are simply suggesting that these women make great friends. You don't have to deal with the usual sexual tension between a male and a female; it is understood from the beginning that the two of you are merely friends.

Most guys, however, are not sure how to deal with the discovery that a woman is in a relationship. In fact, even if they're engaged in incredible conversation with a woman and things appear to be going really well, most guys find a way to end the conversation within thirty seconds once she mentions her boyfriend or husband. We used to be like this as well, but we've changed our ways since we started observing Oscar.

Whenever a woman brings up her boyfriend or husband to Oscar, he encourages her to talk about him. Oscar asks questions about him, such as:

> "Oh, how did the two of you meet?"
> "How long have you been dating/married?"
> "Where does he live?"
> "What does he do?"
> "Oh, where is he tonight?"

This really shocks most women who expect that Oscar will want to end the conversation now that they've mentioned their significant other. When a woman mentions her boyfriend or husband, Oscar continues the conversation just as he normally would and proceeds to ask for her contact info. These women are often the most willing to give out their contact info because they realize that Oscar isn't hitting on them!

Guys often tell us that one of their worst experiences is when they're having a great conversation with a woman, but when they ask for her contact info, she replies with something such as:

> "Oh, I'm sorry, but I'm seeing someone."
> "I don't think my boyfriend would like it if I gave you my phone number."
> "I'm sorry, but I have a boyfriend."

Smooth and sincere as always, Oscar will offer up something such as the following response:

> "I wasn't trying to hit on you. You just mentioned that you really like karaoke, and a bunch of friends and I are going to a karaoke bar sometime next week. So I wanted to invite you and your boyfriend to join us."

We've found that a woman will typically respond:

> "Oh, that sounds like a lot of fun. My boyfriend usually works late during the week, but I'd love to join the group."

Next thing you know, you're walking into the karaoke bar with a ravishing redhead by your side – your subconscious vouch for the evening! Every woman in there sees you walking in with her and thinks, "Damn! I'd kill to be her tonight!" Makes you think twice about your qualms about befriending women, doesn't it?

Part II The Nice Guys' Guide™ to Approaching Women

In the "Approaching Women" section of The Nice Guys' Guide to Getting Girls™, we discussed how to convey interest in a conversation, and the importance of not talking about yourself. In Part II of The Nice Guys' Guide 2™, we will offer further advice on maintaining a conversation with a beautiful woman, meeting women at parties and social gatherings, and complimenting women, that we at The Nice Guys' Institute™ have discovered since our last book.

Chapter 4 – The Nice Guys' Guide™ to Maintaining a Conversation

In previous books in *The Nice Guys' Guide*™ Series, we provided a roadmap for successful introductory conversation between a male and a female. Although we provided a sample introductory conversation equipped with analysis, guys often tell us that they have trouble keeping a conversation going. They tell us that they will often get a woman engaged in conversation, but then they don't know what to do or say next. So, they find themselves forced to prematurely end the conversation before they have a good reason to get the woman's contact info. With that in mind, we at The Nice Guys' Institute™ have learned of several strategies that you can employ to keep a conversation going. By using these, you should be able to keep any conversation going for at least ten minutes – just long enough to get a woman's contact info!

1. Compliment and follow-up. Use this when a woman mentions something that she is proud of. Compliment the object or event and then ask a follow-up question about it:

> Female: "I ran my first half-marathon last weekend."
>
> Male: "Wow! What a great accomplishment! You must be so proud! What got you interested in running a half-marathon?"

> Female: "I got this tattoo after my grandfather passed away."
>
> Male: "Wow, that's really great that you did that to honor him. What made you decide to get the tattoo?"

2. Respond to a general question with another question. Sometimes a woman will pose a general question, such as asking if you've heard about something in the news. If you can't think of anything insightful to say in response, then reply by asking her a question or two about it. If she brought it up, then it's probably something of interest to her that she can talk about at-length:

> Female: "Did you hear that every doctor in the city is walking out on the job?"
>
> Male: "Yeah, I can't believe it. Can you remember this ever happening before? What do you think will happen?"

> Female: "Did you know that Jerry Springer is thinking about running for governor?"
>
> Male: "No, I hadn't heard that. Do you think he'll actually go through with it?"

3. Transition to a new topic using something she just said. Often, you'll ask a question and get only a brief response, thus ending your discussion about that

topic. However, the woman will often mention something in her answer that you can use to start another discussion. Picking up on these cues and transitioning the conversation appropriately is essential to making this approach work:

> Male: "Yeah, I have a pretty good base tan. How about you – are you naturally this dark?"
> Female: "No, I got my tan when I was down in Bermuda."
> Male: "Oh, wow, Bermuda – how was it?"

> Male: "That is a really pretty necklace; I've never seen a design like that before."
> Female: "Thank you. I got it when I was in New Mexico."
> Male: "I've never been to New Mexico. What was it like?"

4. Ask how she thinks or feels about something. Many times during a conversation, a woman will mention something that she heard about that you either know very little about or don't really have anything insightful to add. An easy way to advance the conversation is to ask how she thinks or feels about that:

> Female: "I heard on the radio today that the governor wants to raise the sales tax rate."
> Male: "I heard about that. What do you think about his decision?"

> Female: "My daughter's thinking about going back to school. Again."
> Male: "Wow, I didn't know that. How do you feel about that?"

5. Ask for clarification. This technique is best used to demonstrate that you are paying attention to and interested in what she's talking about. If a woman

is telling a story that you're having trouble following, stop and ask her a question about one of the details in the story. This will ensure that you stay on track and show her that you are in fact listening.

> Female: "And then my phone rang while I was sitting there on the side of the road. And I wasn't sure if it was my dad calling back or the tow truck."
>
> Male: "I'm sorry, I'm not sure I got all that. Did you say that your car broke down first or that you got the call from your dad first?"

> Female: "And then Rachel called me up and told me the news which, of course, I'd already heard firsthand from Josh."
>
> Male: "Wait a minute, I'm a little confused. Is Rachel Josh's current girlfriend or his ex-girlfriend?"

6. Ask for more details. This is one of the most basic tactics for maintaining a conversation. When a woman tells you something, simply ask for more details about the event:

> Female: "I can't believe I went bungee jumping yesterday!"
>
> Male: "I've always thought about trying it. How difficult was it to make yourself jump?!"

> Female: "I went skiing for the first time today."
>
> Male: "Oh, I remember my first time skiing; how did you like it?"

7. Show that you understand how something made her feel. When women communicate, they will often discuss an event for the purpose of relaying their emotions. However, they usually won't come right out and tell you how they're feeling. This is very unfortunate for men. Women, on the other hand, can

somehow instinctively tell how another woman is feeling. When you hear two women talking, you will often hear one say, "Oh, I can see how that would make you feel unfulfilled." If you can be one of the rare men who picks up on the fact that a woman is trying to communicate her feelings, women everywhere will want to be around you. Initially, it might be difficult for you to read a woman's emotional state and remark, "Oh, I can see how that would make you feel unfulfilled." However, a good way to test your instincts to see if you're right is to ask a question:

> Female: "He asks me to do the most menial tasks. I have a freaking college degree, for crying out loud."
> Male: "Sounds like you're feeling very unfulfilled at work, huh?"

> Female: "My boss told me today that when I switch departments at the end of the month, he's not backfilling my role."
> Male: "And so that made you feel unimportant?"

8. Ask for an example. Because of the discrepancies between the way that males and females communicate, we men often don't really understand what a woman is saying. Don't be afraid to ask for an example as clarification:

> Female: "You know, when you're feeling sad, and you think it's one thing, but it's actually another?"
> Male: "I think I know what you mean. Can you give me an example?"

> Female: "Do you know that shade of blue, not quite cyan but not quite teal?"
> Male: "Is there something in the room that's similar in color?"

9. Ask how she managed. When a woman is telling you about a tough time in her life, compliment her perseverance and ask how she coped with the situation:

> Female: "My mom was sick for two of the years that I was in college."
>
> Male, *compassionately*: "That must have been really tough for you. How did you manage?"

> Female: "When my husband passed away, I had an eight-month-old daughter and no job. It was tough, but I seem to have made it through the worst of it."
>
> Male, *sympathetically*: "Wow, I imagine that that must have been really difficult for you. You're a real survivor. How did you find the time to work part-time while going to school and raising a daughter?"

10. Ask why. When a woman offers up an opinion that she's heard, ask why that is the case.

> Female: "A lot of people are opposed to the tax cut."
>
> Male: "Hmmm... I didn't realize that. Do you know what their reasoning is?"

> Female: "They're talking about recalling the governor."
>
> Male: "Do you know why so many people are disappointed with him when his approval rating was so high just six months ago?"

Don't try to solve a woman's problems

When guys have a problem, we consult our friends in search of advice. The sooner our friends can offer us advice, the sooner we can resolve the problem and get on with our lives. When a woman is discussing a problem, however, she wants exactly the opposite. She merely wants someone to listen to her so that she can get the problem off of her chest.

Herein lies a fundamental difference between men and women in conversation: When women are discussing a problem, they don't want the listener to offer up a solution. Guys frequently make the mistake of trying to solve a woman's problem and then end the conversation or change the subject. While you probably think it's a good idea to help a woman solve her problems since you're used to serving that function for your male friends, you couldn't be more wrong. Although you'd expect the woman to be gracious and thankful when you help solve her problems, your attempt to solve her problems will only frustrate her and create a new problem in turn: resentment toward you. When you offer up solutions to a woman's problems, you're sending her the message that:

> "I don't want to sit here and listen to you talk about your problems. The quicker I can offer a solution, the quicker I can go back to watching the game."

Obviously, Nice Guys like us don't want the women in our lives to think that we're trying to shut them up. So how can we let women air their problems without overstepping our bounds? Here are a couple of examples of what *not* to say, followed by examples of what you should say:

Female: "He asks me to do the most menial tasks. I have a freaking college degree, for crying out loud."

Male (*wrong response*): "Well, just tell him that you have a college degree, and you expect to be doing more challenging work. Or better yet, quit the job."

Female: "Ugh, I'm just so frustrated! Are you even listening to me?!"

Female: "He asks me to do the most menial tasks. I have a freaking college degree, for crying out loud."

Male (*correct response*): "It sounds like you're feeling very unfulfilled at work."

Female: "Yes, exactly! Like today, he put a bunch of envelopes on my desk and asked me to file them. Does he think I'm his secretary or something?!"

Female: "My boss told me today that when I switch departments at the end of the month, he's not backfilling my role."

Male (*wrong response*): "So just switch departments and don't look back. Who cares?"

Female, *frustrated*: "You really don't get it, do you? How would you feel if you left your job and they didn't hire anyone to replace you?"

Female: "My boss told me today that when I switch departments at the end of the month, he's not backfilling my role."

Male (*correct response*): "I take it that made you feel insignificant?"

Female: "Yeah. I've worked my tail off for him the last few years, and this is how he repays me? By telling me that my job isn't important enough to maintain after I'm gone?"

Another big mistake guys make is telling a woman how she should feel about something or, worse yet, trying to minimize her feelings. Often guys will do this by trying to steal the limelight from the woman and relating her problem back to their own experiences. *Bad idea.* When a woman is upset or bothered about something, what she wants above all is for someone to listen to her and show support for her feelings. She wants someone to recognize how she feels and approve of those feelings. Let's revisit the previous examples and examine responses that minimize the woman's feelings or tell her how she should feel. See how much of yourself you hear in these responses:

Female: "He asks me to do the most menial tasks. I have a freaking college degree, for crying out loud."

Male (*wrong response, questions her feelings*): "Why are you upset about that? I had to do menial tasks for a year when I started."

Male (*wrong response, minimizes her feelings*): "You shouldn't let it bother you. Just do the work, and I'm sure you'll get to do more exciting stuff eventually."

Male (*wrong response, tells her how to feel*): "Don't make such a big deal about this. You should be grateful that you even have a job."

Female: "My boss told me today that when I switch departments at the end of the month, he's not backfilling my role."

Male (*wrong response, questions her feelings*): "Why do you even care? You're moving on to a better job."

Male (*wrong response, minimizes her feelings*): "Don't be upset about that. At least you've got another job. I hate my job, and I can't find another one. "

Male (*wrong response, tells her how to feel*): "Just be happy that you're leaving your boss behind and moving on to better things."

When you try to solve a woman's problems or disapprove of her feelings, you will discourage her from talking to you and encourage her to find someone else to share her feelings with and provide her with emotional support. Remember, women bond through feelings and emotions, and if you're not providing an adequate outlet for your wife's or girlfriend's emotions, then she may turn elsewhere, potentially even to another man. If the other guy is open and receptive and encourages her to share her feelings without criticizing her, then the two of them will start to connect, which could spell the end of your relationship.

The more supportive you are of a woman's feelings, the more she'll want to share things with you. This is absolutely essential if you want to deepen and strengthen your relationship. If you are not supportive of her feelings and some other guy is, then there's a good chance that you'll end up losing her and find yourself back on page one of this book!

We have seen so many men at parties or social gatherings stand in the corner by themselves or sit with a group of guys, clearly missing out on a great opportunity to meet a dozen women very easily in one evening. If you're thinking, "been there, done that," you're in luck. As part of our effort to help you put your wallflower days behind you, we offer you the following guidelines, which should help you figure out what to do the next time you're invited to a party or social gathering:

1. If a female is hosting the party, bring her something.

We've found that most women really love to receive a bottle of wine, perhaps because there's something about wine that implies a bit of class and maturity on your part. It doesn't even have to be an expensive bottle; Oscar often walks in with a $7 bottle of red wine from the grocery store, and women love it (though we're sure by now you realize that women love everything Oscar does)! If it's a backyard cookout hosted by a female friend of yours, call or e-mail her to ask if you can bring anything. Oscar will swing by the grocery store on the way over and buy a pre-made side dish for a few bucks. A simple gesture like this can have tremendous payback in terms of gratitude.

Once you're in the door and have handed the hostess a token of your appreciation, the socializing begins. Don't psych yourself out about this. Parties and social gatherings were designed to help you relax and have fun. In fact, the greatest thing about a party is that that you shouldn't have to stress over initiating conversation. There's one foolproof opening line that you can use over and over again at parties and social gatherings. You can even use the same line on other women who have already witnessed you use it that evening without sounding like a broken record (unless you already used it on them, of course!). Without further ado, we present you the line that just might change your life:

Chapter 5 – The Nice Guys' Guide™ to Parties, Social Gatherings, and Other Group Settings

In previous books in *The Nice Guys' Guide*™ Series, we have suggested that one of the most inviting ways to meet women is at parties and other social gatherings. This is true regardless of your age. We have found that it's extremely easy to meet women at everything from keg parties to backyard cookouts to professional cocktail parties. The reason it is so easy to meet women in these environments is that you're not bothering them. When women attend a party or a social gathering, they expect to meet new people. Heck, they might even be there solely for that purpose. Additionally, they assume that you must be a decent guy since you were invited there and thus know the host. While women will most likely reach this assumption on their own, it's still up to you to prove that you're a decent human being. This shouldn't be that difficult, but apparently it is for many guys.

2. "So how do you know <host's name>?"

When you meet women at a bar or at a bookstore, there's never one universal line that is guaranteed to start a conversation. At a party, however, you can use this line on any woman, and you'll almost always find that she'll talk to you. And, of course, don't forget to use the standard guidelines that we presented in previous books in *The Nice Guys' Guide*™ Series for having a great conversation, such as making eye contact, asking follow-up questions, and offering up short responses about yourself.

The great thing about a party or social gathering is that not only do you have a guaranteed opening line, but that one opening line can facilitate great conversation. For example, the woman will usually respond with something such as she went to school with the host, works with the host, knows him from their childhood, grew up next door to him, or took an acting class with him last year. Regardless of the response, it will provide you with great potential for follow-up questions. For example, if they're childhood friends, you can follow-up with,

> "Oh, where did you two grow up?"
> "Did you live there your entire childhood?"
> "Where else have you lived?"
> "Do your parents still live there?"
> "Do you have siblings? Where are they now?"

Of course, don't ask these questions in rapid succession. Rather, it's best to ask a question, wait for a response, offer a short follow-up remark about yourself, and ask another question, as we have instructed in previous books in *The Nice Guys' Guide*™ Series. You can also refer to the Appendix for more great questions to ask when you first meet a woman.

3. Don't forget to introduce yourself at some point during the conversation.

And be sure to remember her name! We often witness guys at parties struggle to remember women's names, or anything about them for that matter. The great thing about a party is, as we said, you can easily meet four, five, six, even a dozen women in one evening. However, there's also a downside to this: It's nearly impossible to remember every woman's name, much less anything else you've learned about them.

Whenever we're at a party, we always look for a pen and a napkin lying around. After we've chatted with a woman for ten minutes or so, we head into the bathroom with the pen and napkin and jot down her name and a few of the things she told me. This is extremely important at a party – much more so than at a bar. The second you get out of that bathroom, you're likely to wind up talking with someone else. You certainly don't want your previous conversation to have been all for naught simply because you couldn't remember her name, or worse yet, confused her with another woman!

4. Don't be afraid to enter ongoing conversations.

Your mother may have taught you not to interrupt other people while they're speaking, but that doesn't mean that you shouldn't walk up to a group of people that is having a conversation and include yourself in the circle. Quite the contrary. Doing so is actually essential to expanding your horizons, abandoning your social anxiety, and meeting new women. Unfortunately, though, many guys don't seem to have figured this out yet.

Frequently, we'll see a group of people – often a group comprised of both men and women – standing around at a party. For some reason, many guys will walk right past this group and sit down by themselves, go hold up the wall, or walk up to some guy they know and start chatting with him. Meanwhile, they're missing a golden opportunity to meet three new women!

Entering a group conversation at a party is one of the greatest and most convenient ways to meet multiple women in a brief amount of time. You simply can't do this at a bar. If you see a group of people conversing at a bar, the odds are pretty high that they all know each other and will wonder why some strange guy randomly joined their conversation. At a party or social gathering, on the other hand, the odds are decent that a few of the people in this group just met each other. Even if they are all friends, they usually won't mind someone else joining them since you must be friends with the host as well!

With this in mind, you can walk up and participate in any group conversation at a party, and you will most likely be welcome. Of course, use basic rules of etiquette: Don't interrupt someone else mid-sentence, and don't barge in with a rude or off-the-wall comment. Simply wait until there's an opportunity in the conversation for you to add something. Or, if there's a lull in the conversation, just look at everyone and say, "So how do you guys know <host's name>?" This icebreaker can prove quite useful for meeting a few new women. My friend Brooke talks about her favorite way to meet guys at a party:

> "The best way to meet me at a party is to join in on a group conversation. Now, don't interrupt me if I'm standing there talking to one of my girlfriends one-on-one. That's a real pain. But if I'm in a group of people talking about something, usually not everyone in the group knows each other that well! So feel free to jump in and join the conversation. That's the best way to meet guys at a party!"

5. Meet everyone at a party

Since you'll generally find that the groups of people standing around are comprised of both men and women, you might have realized that you'll inevitably wind up meeting guys as well as women. When we're at a party or social gathering, we try to meet everyone there, guys and women alike. We don't even mind meeting women who are there with guys. In our experience, the most important thing is to meet a few new people early in the evening when you first get to the party. This includes single women, guys, and women who are there with guys as well. As the evening progresses and more and more people arrive, you will inevitably be introduced to these newcomers since you have been chatting with their friends. We often find that a beautiful woman will be standing there talking to someone whom we just met earlier in the evening, which gives us a good excuse to introduce ourselves. For instance, consider a party one of The Nice Guys™ was at just last weekend:

> I noticed a man and a woman standing in the living room early in the evening. I immediately walked up, introduced myself, and learned that they're husband and wife, David and Janice. I chatted with them for a few minutes and then moved on to meet some other people. In retrospect, introducing myself to them was the best decision I made all night!

> About an hour later, a beautiful Puerto Rican woman walked in. She was a mirror image of Jennifer Lopez, and I later found out that her friends call her J-Lo for this very reason! She was so beautiful that even I would have been intimidated approaching her (and these days that rarely happens). However, I didn't have to approach her.

As luck would have it, J-Lo happened to be a long-time friend of Janice and David's. When I saw her chatting with Janice and David fifteen minutes later, I walked right up. It was great because Janice immediately motioned to me, "John, I want you to meet my friend Bianca. Bianca, this is John."

Next thing I knew, I was standing there chatting with Janice, David, and Bianca. Bianca and I hit it off well, and Janice and David ended up leaving the party. After they left, Bianca and I chatted for another twenty minutes and exchanged e-mail addresses. Just think, simply by taking a few minutes early in the evening to make small talk with Janice and David, I ended up meeting the most beautiful woman there! Sure, some of it may have been the result of luck and good timing, but my success that evening had almost everything to do with the fact that I took the initiative and socialized with total strangers of both sexes.

Now that you have learned the keys to meeting women at parties and social gatherings, we have dedicated the rest of this chapter to addressing a few of your most commonly asked questions about parties, social gatherings, and interacting with groups of people.

QUESTION: I was at a party the other day and there was a group of us standing around talking. Then suddenly this one guy changed the subject and started talking about some really depressing topics that no one really wanted to hear about. Everyone had been in a great mood and suddenly everyone, at least in this social circle, seemed really down after listening to him. What's the best way to handle a situation like this?

ANSWER: We, too, have been in situations like this plenty of times. The best thing to do is to gracefully exit that group of people. Say something like:

> "Oh, if you guys will excuse me, I've got to use the bathroom" or

> "If you guys will excuse me, I'm going to go grab another drink."

We have found that when we do this, quite often another person or two in the circle will go with us. They'll say something like, "Oh, yeah. Me too," and go with us just to get out of there. What we've learned not to do is to pass judgment on the person or try to change the subject. If you do either of those two things, then you may be thought of as rude. This is because there may be other people standing around who do want to discuss this topic.

For instance, at a party we were at recently, the conversation suddenly turned to the topic of parents dying. This appeared to make quite a few people uncomfortable and really brought the mood of the conversation down. Unfortunately, one guy in the group actually made an attempt to change the topic, which would have been great with most of us, but one girl who was standing there had recently dealt with her mother passing away and was very offended that this guy wanted to change the topic of conversation.

While the topic of conversation may be obviously boring or offensive to the majority of the group of people, by changing the topic of conversation, you also might offend someone in the group who honestly wants to discuss that topic. This was the case when this guy tried to change the topic away from death. As we said, the best thing to do is to politely exit the conversation by going to the restroom or getting another drink or some food.

QUESTION: I tend to be highly competitive by nature. This is great for me on the athletic field, but in conversation it often doesn't translate so well. For example, just last night at a party, I ended up in heated discussions on three different occasions. In the first case, I ended up arguing with this guy over who has the better fantasy football team. On the second occasion, I ended up quarreling with this girl over which mall was closer. And in the third case, I ended up bickering with a few people over the derivation of a word. In all three cases, I knew I was right and the other person was wrong. Of course, this didn't seem to go a long way to winning anyone's favor.

I've always behaved this way, but after taking your courses and listening to your audio series, I've started to realize that maybe I need to change my ways. My innate need to always win arguments and always prove myself right, and everyone else wrong, seems to be hurting me socially. What are your thoughts?

ANSWER: It appears that you have come to the correct conclusion on your own. It is unfortunate, but what you say is true of a lot of guys. We tend to be very competitive and argumentative by nature. In fact, quite often we witness guys arguing over the most trivial things. In a lot of these cases, yes, the guys are right. The argument, however, is usually petty and, although the guy feels better about winning the argument, everyone else thinks less of him.

Are we saying never to present your point of view? Not necessarily, but there are a couple of points that we'd like to make. First, if you're talking to a beautiful woman whom you're interested in, then arguing with her really serves no good purpose. She may be dead wrong about how close the mall is, or the derivation of some word, but it really serves no purpose to correct her. Think about it. The last time someone corrected you and rubbed it in your face, did you feel better afterward? Hell, no. You resented the fact that he or she showed you up like that.

If you do feel some overwhelming urge to disagree with people in conversation, then at least try to avoid doing so while in conversation with a beautiful woman. And if you do feel the need to argue with guys, for example, over who has the better fantasy football team, then try to avoid phrases like these:

> "You're so wrong."
> "Oh, I told you I was right."
> "Ha, in your face."
> "You're an idiot!"
> "That's what you get for going to a stupid state school."
> "Chalk another one up for me."

This conversation is, of course, fine when you're hanging out with the guys watching football on a Sunday afternoon. When you're at a social gathering making obnoxious comments like these, however, it will really turn off the women within earshot. There are polite ways to tell someone that he or she is wrong, such as:

> "Actually I'm not sure if that's right. I think that word may be Latin actually, although I'm not positive myself."

Although this statement doesn't provide you with the overwhelming satisfaction of rubbing your victory in someone's face, it is much better used in a social context. It will have much less of a negative effect on the women in the surrounding environment, and it's worth forgoing the opportunity to show up one of your friends if you go home with a beautiful woman's phone number instead!

QUESTION: I witnessed this guy the other night, who made a habit of finishing everyone else's statements. He's what I guess you can call a "know-it-all." For example, no matter what anyone said, he had been there, done that. At one point someone brought up Germany. He immediately responded, "Oh, yeah. I've been to Germany many times," and then started talking about his travels to Germany. Later on, someone mentioned they were an architect. He said, "Oh, yes. I used to work in an architectural firm," and started talking about his job there. At some point, someone mentioned California and he said, "Yes, I grew up on the coast of San Diego," and started talking about all the places he had lived in San Diego. It's like no matter what anyone said, he had to interject the fact that he'd been there, done that, and knew more about the place than anyone else in the conversation. Is this as bad a thing as it looks?

ANSWER: This is definitely as bad as it looks. The larger problem this guy has is his attitude, more so than simply the content of what he's saying. It appears from the way you wrote it that his comments come across in a very arrogant manner, as if he's trying to show everyone up – that he's trying to prove that he's better than them because he's been everywhere they've been and done everything they've done. Unfortunately, arrogance has the opposite effect on people. The more arrogant you are about having done everything and been everywhere, the more you will turn people off and make people *not* want to talk to you.

People enjoy talking about their own experiences – where they've been, and what they've done. When you constantly interject by telling them that you've been there too and you've done that too, especially in an arrogant manner, you're trying to one-up them. What you're saying to the person, in essence, is, "Anything you can do, I can do better." Or "I'm better than you," which will make anyone not want to talk to you.

This naturally leads to the follow-up question: What if you honestly have lived in San Diego, or been to Germany, or worked in an architectural firm? Are you allowed to share these things with other people as they arise in conversation? Absolutely, but there is a very polite way to do so. Look at these examples:

> Female: "I'm an architect actually."
> Male: "Oh, wow! I used to work for an architectural firm. How do you like it?"
>
> Female: "Yeah, I got it on my trip to Germany a couple of years ago."
> Male: "Oh, I love Germany. What did you think of it?"
>
> Female: "Yeah, I used to be stationed out in San Diego."
> Male: "Really? I actually grew up there. How long were you there for?"

Notice how in each of these examples, the male interjected and offered up a fact about himself, but didn't do so in a conceited and arrogant manner; he certainly wasn't trying to show the woman up. Additionally, he made sure to ask a follow-up question, to show that he was, in fact, more interested in what she had to say then continuing to ramble on about himself.

Approaching women in groups is one of the most important techniques to have, if you're ever going to be successful dating women. Because it is so important, we at The Nice Guys' Institute™ are making every effort to research more and more ways for guys to easily approach women in groups. Please visit www.TheNiceGuysGuide.com to learn about our latest findings.

Visit the site often as we are constantly updating it with new content, including downloadable e-books and e-reports, audio tapes and CDs, and video cassettes and DVDs packed with our latest discoveries. We also maintain information on our web site about upcoming coaching sessions, course offerings, and speaking engagements. Additionally, we encourage readers to e-mail us, either through our web site, or at TheNiceGuys@TheNiceGuysGuide.com. Finally, please also come by and sign up for our free newsletter to receive the hottest tips to help nice guys like you make themselves more attractive to women WITHOUT turning into jerks!

Chapter 6 – The Nice Guys' Guide™ to Compliments

In previous books in *The Nice Guys' Guide*™ Series, we stressed the importance of complimenting women. We explained the basics of how to compliment women, gave examples of what to compliment women on, discussed the importance of Third-Party Compliments, and talked about the types of compliments to avoid.

Nevertheless, we continue to receive many questions about complimenting women. So we wanted to offer up some more tips on how to properly compliment women:

1. Learn to use non-physical compliments

A lot of guys have told us that they understand how to appropriately compliment a woman's jewelry, accessories, and physical beauty, but they often have difficulty conveying to a woman that they like her as a person. We thus want to offer some brief insight to men about how to offer up non-physical compliments in the appropriate manner. Please keep in mind that the key to *any* compliment is that you are genuine and sincere. You must always utter a compliment confidently – and with eye contact. With that in mind, here are some examples of how to compliment women in a non-physical manner:

"It must have taken a lot of courage to give up that great job and go back to school. I'm really impressed that you were willing to make that sacrifice."

"You're such a determined person. Even when everyone in your family told you that you'd never get into a good law school, you studied your tail off for the LSAT. And now you're going to Harvard Law School. I can't tell you how impressed I am by your determination!"

"You always maintain such a positive attitude. That's why I love spending time with you. No matter how bad my day has been, I know that I always have your beautiful smiling face to look forward to." [*Note: This uses both a physical and non-physical compliment.*]

"Wow! You have such an incredible voice! Why haven't I ever heard you sing before?"

"I have so much respect for your work as a nurse. It takes a certain kind of person to work twelve hour shifts that require her to stand on her feet all day long in such an intense environment. Nursing is one of the most important and challenging professions there is, and I really respect you for entering that field."

"I think it's incredible that you're able to hold down such a challenging job while raising two kids."

"I appreciate you taking the time to show me around town and introduce me to such great people. You've really alleviated my stress about moving to a new city and made me feel so welcome here."

"I just wanted you to know that you are an absolutely amazing person. I have such a great time whenever we're together, and I'm really glad that you're a part of my life."

A final word of advice: These are such great compliments that they shouldn't just be reserved for women whom you're dating! If you come across someone – male or female – in your daily interactions worthy of such a compliment, take ten seconds out of your day to relay the message. You'll brighten up that person's day and quite possibly your own! In fact, whenever we are feeling blue or are simply having a bad day, we make it a point to compliment others. Seeing the reaction of another person when we pay him or her a sincere compliment never fails to lift our spirits and build our confidence!

2. Use the person's name in the compliment

When you're complimenting someone, saying the person's name makes the compliment that much more personal and sweeter to hear. Oscar always makes it a point to do this:

"Hey, that's a really pretty sweater you're wearing, Gina."

> "Thanks for taking the time to help me out. You're always so considerate, Susan."

> "I can't believe you painted this, Rachel! You're incredibly talented."

3. Tell her she's the best in the crowd

Another great way to compliment a woman is to show her how special she is by telling her that she is the best in the crowd. For instance, we enjoy turning to a woman who has accompanied one of us somewhere and saying:

> "Wow, you are by far the most exquisitely dressed woman in the room. Aren't I lucky to be with you!"

4. Make eye contact while complimenting

Another rule of thumb that we learned from observing Oscar is to make eye contact when you relay a compliment and offer up a smile afterward. Many guys look away when complimenting a woman, most likely because doing so makes them nervous, and it's difficult to look into someone's eyes when you're nervous. Unfortunately for these guys, a compliment tends to lose its power and luster when you fail to make eye contact. A sincere, confident man will look a woman directly in the eye when complimenting her.

5. Personalize your compliments

Oscar has a knack for complimenting people in very specific and personal terms and, based on women's reactions, it is obvious that this means far more to a woman than a generic compliment. For example, Oscar rarely says:

> "That's a really pretty sweater."

Instead, he'll make eye contact and say something like:

"That's a really pretty sweater. I like the way it matches your eyes, Olivia."

Instead of saying:

"I like your earrings."

Oscar will say:

"Those are really pretty earrings, Megan. I like the way they sparkle in the moonlight."

Instead of merely offering up:

"I have a lot of respect for you,"

Oscar will take the time to convey why he has respect for the woman he's addressing:

"I have a lot of respect for the way you moved across the country by yourself to chase your dream of being an actress. Your independence and determination really impress me, Judy."

6. Don't forget to use Third-Party Compliments

As presented in previous books in *The Nice Guys' Guide*™ Series, a Third-Party Compliment praises someone who is not present at the moment. It's easy to get so caught up in complimenting the person to whom you are talking that you forget about the power of Third-Party Compliments. Rather than repeating what we have said about Third-Party Compliments in previous books, we'll simply remind you that you and the person you're talking to aren't the only two people in the world, so remember to dish out those Third-Party Compliments!

7. Make your compliments believable

Additionally, make sure that the compliments you use sound believable and sincere. It would seem a bit odd (and creepy), for instance, if you told a woman whom you've known for less than three minutes that she's the most amazing person you've ever met. While this is a flattering compliment for someone you're dating, a woman you've just met will probably assume you're only saying that because you want to sleep with her, which will scare the woman away ninety-nine percent of the time. Therefore, when you first meet a woman, use fairly simple compliments. For instance, consider complimenting the woman in question on jewelry or other accessories that are easily noticeable.

8. If you aren't one to compliment people regularly, begin to do so slowly

Sincerity can be a difficult thing to convey, particularly if you – like most guys – aren't prone to complimenting others. If you're not proficient in complimenting, keep in mind two rules of thumb. First, pace yourself. If you suddenly start complimenting everyone you know all of the time, people will wonder what's going on and question your sincerity. When we first started, we tried to merely offer up one compliment to everyone whom we engaged in a conversation during the day. If we saw someone later in the day, we wouldn't offer up a second compliment. Instead, we waited until the next day to offer her (or him) an additional compliment.

Because we didn't dive in headfirst and start complimenting everyone all of the time, people frequently praised each of us for our changes. Our friends and colleagues would say things like:

"Wow, I enjoy being around you so much more than I used to. You're much more upbeat about everything, and you always make me feel great whenever I'm around you. You've really changed for the better."

While people realized that we were changing for the better, no one questioned our motives or our sincerity since it was a gradual, honest change.

Second, we learned from watching Oscar that the key to ensure that people don't wonder whether you have some ulterior motive is to compliment a person regardless of his or her gender. Whenever Oscar compliments other men, his comments are always fairly benign. He'll often say things such as:

"Hey, cool shoes – are they new?" or

"Hey, man – I really like that sweater. Can I ask where you got it?"

Because Oscar compliments men as well as women, no one doubts his sincerity. But if you suddenly start complimenting women all of the time without uttering a kind word to any of your male friends, people are likely to question your motives.

9.   Avoid awkward silence after a compliment

We've all seen a movie or television show where some guy tells the woman he's seeing that he loves her, and for some reason, the entire relationship suddenly crumbles because she's not sure how to respond. OK, maybe we've actually seen more where the woman tells the man that she loves him, and he flees. Either way, it's not a pretty scene. Whether you're contemplating telling someone that you love her or just that you think she looks beautiful, you've probably feared that that compliment could be awkward, or overwhelm her.

Nobody wants to be *that guy*, which probably explains why men frequently ask me how to avert the awkward silence that often ensues after they compliment a woman. With a hint of despair in their voices, these men complain:

> "Often when I compliment a woman, she can't figure out what to say after I relay the compliment. And then we're both standing there in an awkward silence. It almost makes me not want to compliment her or anyone else. How do I avoid this awkward silence after a compliment?"

If you feel uncomfortable complimenting women or you often find yourself in a state of awkward silence after you've complimented a woman, then follow up your compliment with a question. For instance, consider adding a question to some examples from earlier in the chapter:

> "Hey, that's a really pretty sweater, Gina. Can I ask where you got it?"

> "Thanks for taking the time to help me out. You're always so considerate, Susan. How do you always manage to find time to help others?"

> "I can't believe you painted this, Rachel! You're incredibly talented. How long have you been painting?"

10. Learn how to accept compliments

Now that you're paying a lot of compliments, you will inevitably receive many compliments as well, so make sure you learn how to accept compliments that others pay to you. Oscar is great at this. When someone compliments him, Oscar simply smiles and says something like:

"Thank you so much," or

"Thank you. That means a lot to me."

If you feel uncomfortable merely thanking someone for complimenting you, then follow up with a comment about the item in question:

"Thank you for noticing. I just bought these shoes last week."

"Thank you. I bought this watch in Italy a few years ago."

Whatever you do, don't reject the compliment, responding with comments such as, "Oh, who? Me? Nah." When you reject a compliment, you exhibit a lack of self-confidence, which tends to be quite a turn-off. Moreover, when you reject a compliment, you make the person feel bad and deter him or her from paying you future compliments. And who wants to do that?

11. Never tie a compliment to a favor

Now a couple of "don'ts" regarding compliments: *Never* tie a compliment to a favor. One of us used to work with a guy who was known in the office for doing this. You always knew when he wanted something because he would walk up to you, ask how you were doing, and pay you a compliment. Because he only did this when he wanted you to do some work for him, he earned himself a really bad reputation in the office as an insincere ass-kisser who only paid attention to others when it would benefit him. In fact, after witnessing the impact that this behavior had on his reputation, we now make it a point to *not* compliment someone when we're asking a favor of him or her. We don't want anyone to even accidentally confuse our positive attitude for a subtle attempt to coax him or her into doing us a favor. We want people to realize that we're naturally upbeat and caring people who don't expect anything in return. Trust us, this genuine caring attitude goes a long way.

12. Don't mimic others' compliments

Another "don't": Don't mimic compliments. That's not to say that you shouldn't compliment someone who compliments you, but be original for goodness sake!

You see, we know this guy named Josh who epitomizes exactly how one should *not* return a compliment. Every time someone compliments Josh, he repeats the compliment back to the person, though on occasion he'll add a "too" or "as well" to the comment just for the sake of variety. For instance, if you tell Josh that you like his shoes, he'll tell you that he likes your shoes. Josh may actually like your shoes, but because his comment mimics yours, he tends to sound insincere. As my friend Alyssa explained,

> "When I compliment Josh, I tend to feel like I'm talking to a parrot. Some of my girlfriends and I were talking the other day about how Josh receives compliments. I had thought it was just me, but all of my girlfriends said that he does the same thing with them as well. We started calling him 'Parrot Josh,' but then we felt bad. It just seems like he isn't capable of paying someone a sincere compliment. Don't get me wrong, I'm sure that he means well; it's just a bit pathetic."

So what's the moral of the story? While you should make a point of complimenting others – men and women alike – be original with the words and compliments you use. If you want to sound sincere and be taken seriously when you're returning a compliment, select something else about that person to compliment. In other words, if someone tells you that she really likes your sweater, don't tell her that you really like her sweater – unless, of course, you want her to reply with "Polly want a cracker?"

Chapter 7 – The Nice Guys' Guide™ to Reassurance

In previous books in *The Nice Guys' Guide*™ Series, we explained the importance of reassuring women, stressed the importance of sincerity when being a Nice Guy, and underscored how not to be a doormat, or the "nice guy" whom women walk all over. Guys often tell us, however, that we didn't provide enough instruction on exactly *how* to reassure women. They say that while we appropriately explained women's cries for reassurance, we didn't explain how to handle them. So, for those guys who need a little reassurance on the topic of reassuring women, we will elaborate a little.

It seems like every guy who has ever had a girlfriend or wife has been asked the dreaded question at some point. No, we're not talking about the ominous "do you want to meet my parents?" While the answer to that question is fairly simple – you'll inevitably say, "Yes, of course" while you're really wondering what you've just committed yourself to – the question of which we speak is a much trickier one – one that guys tend to think cannot possibly have a correct answer.

That's right. We're referring to your significant other's questions regarding your perception of her body. Guys often tell us that their wives or girlfriends ask them, "Do I look fat?" or "Do you think these pants make my butt look big?" Typically, guys follow up by asking us, "How on earth am I supposed to respond to *that*?!?"

Before responding, we suggest that you focus less on what the woman is asking and more on *why* she might be asking you this question. A lot of guys will ask us, "Is this her cry for reassurance?" The answer? "Hell, yes."

First of all, notice that women phrase their questions subjectively, never asking:

"Am I fat?" or

"Is my butt big?"

Why do women pose these questions in such a subjective manner? Because they want a subjective answer! This is their cry for reassurance. When a woman asks, "Do I look fat?" what she's really saying is, "I think I've put on some weight. Please, please, PLEASE tell me you still find me attractive!" Women don't want the truth; they simply want the men that they love to tell them that they still look great. They want to know that, despite the fact that they're getting older and their bodies are changing, their men still find them attractive.

Knowing exactly what this dreaded question means should make it a bit easier for you to respond. In fact, while this question may be tricky, there are actually correct and incorrect answers. Here are a few answers that you can choose from to reassure her:

a)   "No, not at all." Simply tell her that she doesn't look like she's gained a pound. White lies are OK. Even if she is gaining a little weight, she will feel so much better if you tell her that she still looks great. If you're comfortable telling a white lie, then she'll love hearing it!

b)   "Honey, you're always beautiful to me." Sometimes honesty – or something close to it – really is the best policy. This answer, from the guy's perspective, both avoids the white lie and allows you to tell her the truth by answering the question that she really wants answered. You still do find her beautiful, and you're providing the reassurance that she craves and needs.

c)   "You know I will always love you no matter what." Here again you avoid telling a white lie. You're not telling her that she hasn't gained weight. You're merely telling her that you will always love her no matter what she looks like, which is very reassuring for anyone to hear.

Now let's look at some incorrect answers:

"Yes, honey, I think you have gained weight."

"Yes, honey, you have definitely put on a few pounds."

"I wish you looked like you did the day we first met."

If you even think about uttering a response like any – or, heaven forbid, all – of these, you will hurt her feelings tremendously. You may also find yourself single again and in need of rereading the entire *The Nice Guys' Guide*™ Series, this time a little more carefully. Please, for the sake of your relationship, choose one of the correct responses that we suggested earlier.

Let's be honest, neither gender ages gracefully. You don't look like you did the day you met her either. However, unlike women, men often don't mind the way they age. In fact, we often take pride in our potbellies, baldness, and newfound hairiness elsewhere on our bodies! Rather than essentially telling your lover to suck it up and "be a man," it is important to recognize that women often don't embrace the aging process as well as men do and to provide them some reassurance along the way.

Don't delude yourself into thinking that you'll only need to reassure women as their bodies change, however. Frequently, guys tell me about women much like the following:

> "There's this girl who I've recently started dating. She always makes comments like, 'Oh, I'm so stupid' or 'I always ask the dumbest questions.' Why does she say things like this? Is this her cry for reassurance?"

Yes, these comments, which reflect the woman's low self-esteem, are indeed cries for reassurance. While her negative self-image might stem from a number of factors in her past as we discussed in *Make Every Girl Want You*™, you can really help her feel a lot better by picking up on her cues for reassurance and responding appropriately. For example, if she says, "Oh, I'm so stupid," respond with something along the lines of:

> "No, you're not. I couldn't believe how much you know about art. You really amazed me when we were walking through the art gallery earlier."

Or, if she says,

"I always ask the dumbest questions,"

you can reassure her by responding:

"No, you're just a really inquisitive, curious person. I'm really impressed by your desire to constantly learn new things."

Part III The Nice Guys' Guide™ to Building Confidence, Multiple Male Orgasms, and the Movies

In Part III of The Nice Guys' Guide™, we will offer further advice on a range of topics that didn't fit neatly into any other section. This includes building your confidence, having multiple orgasms (without losing your erection!), and movie dates, all things that we at The Nice Guys' Institute™ have discovered since our last book.

Chapter 8 – The Nice Guys' Guide™ to Building Confidence

In previous books in *The Nice Guys' Guide*™ Series, we have discussed confidence, why you can't fake it, and the relationship between confidence and your ability to attract women. Yet, time and time again, guys approach us with a hint of insecurity in their voices and say:

> "Women always suggest that confidence is attractive. Nice Guys, you always suggest that confidence is attractive. How do I build confidence? Where can I get some confidence?"

It would be great if Calvin Klein could package up some confidence in a little plastic container for you to spray on yourself whenever you wanted to attract women. But since Calvin Klein isn't quite that sophisticated yet, you're just going to have to read on. Our guess is that by the end of this chapter, you'll feel capable of taking confidence-building measures into your own hands.

Truth be told, confidence comes as a result of success. You can only be genuinely confident about something once you've been successful at it. Back in our pathetic days, we all had very little confidence when we approached women. We suppose that our lack of confidence could be attributed to the fact that we had never had much success at approaching women, so we had no reason to believe this time would be any different. Nowadays, though, we are extremely confident when we approach women. Women sense this confidence, which enhances their attraction to us. I guess you're probably wondering how this 180-degree transformation occurred. The answer, of course, is that we built our confidence through our success at approaching women. We're sure this explanation sounds very circular to you. How did we become successful at approaching women by building the necessary confidence to become successful at approaching women?!

Here's the answer: The key to building confidence is to do so in a step-by-step manner. Suppose we had decided to dive in headfirst and used the mindset that most guys use:

> "Even though I'm pathetic at approaching women, I'm going to try to master everything at once. I'm going to master approaching women, the introductory conversation, getting contacting info, asking women out, and dating simultaneously."

We are almost certain that we would have continued to reign as the King of Pathetic if we had taken this approach. Attempting to master everything at once would have spelled certain doom since making one wrong move at any point in the process could've been lethal for our self-esteem. We may have had a great conversation with a woman and then failed at getting her contact information. Or we may have gotten her contact information, but then she wouldn't return our phone calls. In either case, we would have inevitably considered all of these instances failures, which would have been demoralizing.

So, we instead learned to try to master only one step at a time. Then, as we mastered each step, we became extremely confident about that particular step, which then provided us with the confidence we needed to continue on and succeed at a future step. The first thing we wanted to do was to merely learn how to approach women and engage them in conversation for a few minutes. That's all we wanted to try initially. We decided that no matter how great the conversation went, we wouldn't even ask for her contact info because that might lead to a rejection, which would have destroyed our confidence. We simply wanted to revel in our successes at approaching women in order to build our confidence.

So we simply walked up to women, struck up conversations, tried to make them last for about five to ten minutes, and at the end told them, "I really enjoyed chatting with you. Hopefully I'll see you around," and walked away. And do you know what? The results were amazing!

All of the pressure had disappeared. We were no longer stressing out about asking for contact info and asking women out. We were merely approaching women as genuinely Nice Guys, having great conversations, and ending on a positive note. When we started to realize how easy it was for us to approach women, we became extremely confident. Sure, we knew that not every woman would talk to us, but we knew that on any given night, we would be able to strike up a quality ten-minute conversation with at least a few women throughout the course of the evening. This gave us the confidence we needed to set our next goal – asking for contact info. Our friend Laurie talks about meeting confident guys:

"There's nothing sexier than when a confident guy approaches me and starts talking to me. I can sense it immediately. This guy just feels comfortable talking to women – he exudes confidence. Cause there's nothing worse than the exact opposite: the uncomfortable, stuttering guy who can't think of what to say. But if you're that sexy, confident guy who very confidently strikes up a conversation with me and exudes confidence, then I'm going home with you!"

We decided that because we had become extremely comfortable and confident talking to women, we would start asking for contact info. And you know what? The results were even better than we expected! Because we were approaching women in a confident manner and knew that we could engage many women in a ten-minute conversation, almost all of them were willing to give us their contact info!

At this point, we didn't even bother contacting these women further because we didn't want to risk rejection and find ourselves back at square one. Quickly, our confidence really started to skyrocket. Over a period of a few weeks, we had gone from pathetic, confidence-deficient guys who couldn't converse with a woman if our lives depended on it to guys who felt extremely confident going out at night. We had turned into guys who knew that when they went out at night, they could easily approach a few women throughout the course of the evening, engage them in conversation, and get their contact information.

We recognized at that point that we wouldn't be successful every time, but we knew that our success rate was much higher than it had ever been, and this made our confidence soar. Equipped with plenty of self-esteem, we were finally ready to complete this multi-step confidence-building strategy. When we got a woman's contact info, we would proceed with the rest of the guidelines in the previous books in *The Nice Guys' Guide*™ Series. We would e-mail the woman, build rapport, invite her out on a very casual first date, and take things from there.

Now, we're not suggesting that you should follow our path to a tee. By all means, if you have a great conversation and get a beautiful woman's contact info, feel free to contact her. We're simply telling you what worked for us. Just keep in mind where confidence comes from; confidence isn't something that comes overnight. Rather, it comes from sustained success at something. Recognize that with every additional success you have, you will feel a bit more confident, which in turn will foster further success and boost your confidence even more.

If you find yourself really lost or frustrated, simplify the task at hand. Forget about the stressful requirements of getting a girl's contact info and actually contacting her. Focus instead on simply approaching women and making great conversation. Or, if you're great at approaching women and chatting with them, but you're horrible at first dates, eliminate all of the pressure of the date by not worrying about making a move at the end or even kissing her goodnight. Just plan to have a relaxed evening and enjoy yourself! You'll be surprised – and pleased – how a few successful first dates like that will really build your confidence on future dates.

Chapter 9 – The Nice Guys' Guide™ to Multiple Male Orgasms

In previous books in *The Nice Guys' Guide*™ Series, we have covered various sexual topics at length. Yet a common e-mail that we continue to get is from guys wondering how to last longer! We have actually learned that some guys can have multiple orgasms (yes, like women!), without ever losing their erection. Yes, we're talking about guys who come six or seven times in an hour, all without ever becoming flaccid! Too good to be true? We thought so too, until we heard about it first-hand. Once we found out about this, we *had* to include it in our newest book. Read on!

How many times have you experienced the following scenario:

> "Audrey and I had been having sex for about 10 minutes and I could tell that she was really starting to get turned on. We'd gone through a few different positions. We

started out in missionary. Then we went to doggy style. Now she was riding the hell out of me and I could tell that she was getting really, really close to coming. She probably needed just another minute or two before she could come but I couldn't hold out. The way she was riding me, I just freaking came with the thunder.

Audrey tried to keep riding me but I already started to get limp, so she finally had to stop. I could tell she was really disappointed and I was really disappointed and embarrassed myself. Once again, I couldn't last long enough. I mean, I went 10, maybe 15 minutes but that just wasn't long enough for her. Man, I just come way too quickly."

Listen to what we learned when one of our good friends Judy opened up to us about the European guy she's sleeping with:

"Oh, my God. Logan is the most amazing guy I've ever slept with. I've never seen anything like it. He can last for an hour. But not only that, he comes as many times as I do during sex. Just last night, we made love for an hour. We went through about five or six different positions. In every position, both of us came a time or two.

I've dated some guys before who've lasted long, but they never seemed to be into the sex. It's like they were so focused on making sure that I came, and that they didn't come too soon, so they were never really into it. But not Logan. Logan was just as into it as I was. I've never felt so connected with a guy in my entire life, the way he stared into my eyes and the way he came repeatedly with me. I don't know if this is just a European thing or what. But from now on, I'm only dating European guys!"

Needless to say, we at The Nice Guys' Institute™ were shocked to hear this story. A guy who lasts an hour? A guy who has multiple orgasms? We just couldn't believe it, so we set out on a mission. We started asking everyone we knew about this, and surprisingly enough, we found three guys who claimed to be able to do this. Read on to witness our interviews with Cameron, Gabe, and Bob, three seemingly-normal guys, who are *anything but normal* when it matters the most!

The Nice Guys™: "So what made you become multi-orgasmic?"

Cameron: "Back before I was multi-orgasmic, I had a major, major problem. I came way too soon. Every time I had sex with a girl, or even from oral sex, I would come in like 30 seconds flat. It was embarrassing to me and worse off, I could never bring a woman to an orgasm. I knew for a fact that the women that I was sleeping with just weren't happy with my performance. In fact, back in those days, it was often quite common for me to hear a woman exclaim, 'No, not yet' when I was coming. After a while, things got so out of hand, that I actually felt uncomfortable having sex with women and then I lost my confidence in bed.

At one point, I actually went celibate for two years because it was so embarrassing how quickly I came in bed. Of course, that didn't help much because then when I started having sex again, after that two-year time off, I came even quicker than before. I was coming in like 10-15 seconds. I didn't even make it to 30 seconds. I tried everything I could think of.

I tried using the thickest condoms I could find. Hell, I even tried putting on two condoms, thick lambskin, anything to numb the sensation. That made me last, oh, 45 seconds. I even tried rubbing some of those creams on my penis to desensitize the tip of my penis. And yeah, those worked a little bit. With those, I could last maybe two minutes, sometimes even three, but nothing more. I don't know why. I guess it was just mental because nothing could make me last long enough to make a woman come.

The worst part was when I found out that quite a few of my sexual partners had faked orgasms just to make me feel better. This is when I realized I really needed to change my behavior. The few times I actually thought I had made women come, I hadn't even made them come. It was all an illusion. So I finally sought the help of a sex counselor and she taught me that, rather than focusing on lasting longer, I could instead learn how to come multiple times."

TNG™: "Alright, so how does this work?"

C: "First of all, I don't consider myself really multi-orgasmic like a lot of other guys do, but rather dual-orgasmic because I can have two orgasms without losing my erection. The first time I come, it's just like old times. It happens in about 30 seconds. But with this orgasm, I've learned how to control my PC muscle just at the right time so that when I come, I don't actually ejaculate."

Seeing the confused look on our faces, Cameron continued.

"Yeah, that's right, guys. The secret to a guy having multiple orgasms is that you come, but you don't really come. It still feels just like you come, but you don't actually shoot any fluid out, or maybe you do, but it's usually just a little bit. But don't worry because it still feels great. After I come the first time, I can then go all night long. I can just pound away and pound away and have great sex. Hell, I've gone as long as an hour before coming my second time.

It's after I come the first time without shooting, then I just keep going until I give the woman five or six orgasms. We go through a whole slew of positions, sometimes fast, sometimes slow. And since I've already had my big first orgasm, I'm just all about pleasing the woman for the rest of the time.

Then finally, when I can sense that she's getting tired and she's starting to wear down, I go ahead and shoot my load. In the second orgasm, I just let everything go. My whole body releases and I shoot a freaking bullet. Sometimes I'll try to time this full-blown cum shot with my woman's orgasm so that we can both come at the same time, or other times I'll just let her come five or six times in a row and then I'll shoot my load.

The coolest part about all of this is that I don't lose my erection in between. Now back in the days when I used to come full-blown after 30 seconds, I'd lose my erection and I was toast for an hour. Nowadays though, since I come but I don't really come, after 30 seconds, I don't lose my erection. I can keep going, as I said, for up to an hour without ever having to get it back up again.

It's so funny seeing the puzzled look on some women's faces when they realize that I've come and they start to look disappointed but then I can keep going for up to an hour. After the whole sexual experience, I've had women call me the most incredible names, the most common being 'Superman,' which I have to admit I kind of like. And for the first time in my life, I'm no longer embarrassed in bed. I'm happy to let it all out in the first 30 seconds and I'm extremely confident knowing that I can still go for another 12 rounds, well at least another very long second round."

TNG™: "So was it easy to learn?"

C: "Well, it wasn't the most difficult thing in the world. It definitely took some time and patience and dedication to figure it all out. And yeah, I screwed up plenty of times. There were plenty of times where I continued to shoot my full load after 30 seconds. It was really disappointing at first, but as this happened less and less, it became more and more fun to try. Even nowadays, sometimes if I'm really distracted, if I've had a bad day at work and I can't truly focus during my sexual experience, then yeah, sometimes I'll still come after 30 seconds. Or if it's a woman I don't really want to be with, then I'll just let myself go after 30 seconds. But like 90% of the time now, I go as long as I want to.

TNG™: "Does it still feel as good, even though you don't ejaculate?"

C: "I'll tell you the big obstacle that almost kept me from reaching my full potential was at the beginning, my first orgasm didn't really feel all that good. It felt almost like a half-orgasm, like I was coming but I wasn't really coming. After a few times of doing this, it almost became disappointing, and I didn't really want to continue and try to learn this, but my sex counselor encouraged me to keep trying.

She said that it's frequent in the beginning that the guy often experiences less of an orgasm when he doesn't come but that over time, these orgasms can actually become more powerful then orgasms when you do shoot. Man, am I glad I kept going because nowadays, let me tell you, oh, that first time I come, ummmm, even though I don't shoot my load, it feels better than when I do shoot my load. And the second time I come is just as intense.

By the time I've been going for 30 to 45 minutes, the head of my cock actually starts getting tingly and I can tell that it's about time to shoot the mother-load and whoooo, when I come that second time, oh, I can't even describe it. Thank God I've discovered these techniques. That's all I'm going to say."

After speaking with Cameron, we were so intrigued that we had to find another multi-orgasmic guy. Next we spoke with Gabe:

The Nice Guys™: "So, Gabe, what made you become multi-orgasmic?"

Gabe: "My main problem back in the day was definitely not coming too soon, like a lot of multi-orgasmic guys I've heard of. My problem back then was I just wasn't enjoying sex. I could make it last as long as I wanted to, that wasn't a problem. But the whole time during sex, I was focused on something else, like thinking of Larry Bird. Rather than sitting there and enjoying the experience, I had to sit there and focus so hard on not coming that I couldn't even enjoy sex, and I'm sure my wife could tell.

I mean, she would gaze into my eyes and I couldn't even gaze back into her eyes. I had to stare at the blank white wall in front of us and picture Larry Bird in the three-point contest in tight green shorts. Talk about not enjoying sex, man! And to make it worse, I'm not even a Celtics fan."

After we all recomposed ourselves, after dying from laughter, we asked Gabe to please continue on relating his journey to multi-orgasmicness:

"Well, the cool thing is now that I'm multi-orgasmic, I can actually enjoy sex and I can enjoy coming. I mean, half the times back in my previous life, the cum would just sort of sneak up on me. I'd be like, 'No, no, no. Don't come. Don't come.' It would come and instead of sitting there and getting to enjoy the fact that I was coming inside of a beautiful woman, I was sitting there hating myself, wishing it would go away. Well, nowadays, I know every time I'm going to come I get to enjoy the moment because I'm not actually ejaculating when I'm coming, so I know there's nothing to worry about.

TNG™: "So what got you started on being multi-orgasmic?"

G: "Well, what finally changed my life is when I found a book on the Internet about being multi-orgasmic. As a guy, I didn't know this was possible but I went ahead and read it. I didn't even tell my wife I was reading it. I practiced some of the techniques on my own and then asked my wife to please join me and help me out. Man, was she in for a surprise. It has changed both of our lives. And, you know, I can't even remember which book it was. If I remember, I'll let you guys know.

Now when my wife and I make love, I usually wait about five or ten minutes before I come the first time. A lot of times I'll try and time it with my wife's first orgasm, but I make sure to focus and make sure that I don't come with this orgasm, that I don't ejaculate at all. But man, does it still feel great! My whole body still feels like I'm coming. I feel like liquid's shooting out of me. I know my face gets flushed and my heart rate increases. It still feels just like I'm coming but I'm not coming. Then after that first one, I go on and I usually have between seven to ten orgasms, usually somewhere about two, three, maybe five minutes apart from each other."

TNG™: "You have got to be kidding us."

G: "No, not at all. I'm just like my wife now. You should hear us having sex. It's like a freaking circus in there. We both spend like 45 minutes just yelling at each other. She's coming. I'm coming. She's coming. I'm coming. We're both coming. Every two, three, five minutes, one of us is coming. It's out of control. Then when we're finally both getting tired, we just stop having sex. Sometimes then I go ahead and ejaculate but a lot of times I don't even bother to ejaculate at all.

And you know what? It doesn't bother me one bit. I've actually found that when I come seven to ten times without even ejaculating, I'm not even tired afterward. I feel great. I feel like my wife. I feel revived and full of energy instead of needing to sleep and eat, like most guys do after sex. But the great thing is I don't feel like I haven't come. I mean, I still feel like my body's released all of that sexual energy that it's needed to. I don't feel the least bit horny. I don't feel like there's any sperm pent up in me. I'm not sure how my body's getting rid of it or if I'm just carrying around tons of tons of sperm in my sac. I don't know what's going on, but all I know is I don't even feel a need to ejaculate anymore."

TNG™: "So does it always last this long? Every time you have sex?"

G: "Well, sometimes it does. Sometimes my wife and I go all night long. Well, not really all night long. But 45 minutes to an hour. But then others times, my wife and I are both tired. And yeah, we still both want each other. But we just don't have the energy to go for 45 minutes.

So at those times, we'll just have sex for maybe five, ten, fifteen minutes. We'll each come once. I won't even bother ejaculating. We'll just each come once and call it a night and we still both feel great. The greatest part is I have control over my sex life like never before, and so does my wife."

TNG™: "So was learning how to be multi-orgasmic difficult?"

G: "No, not at all, especially since I'm a well-conditioned athlete. I played football in college, so I'm used to running wind sprints and two-a-days. Compared to what Coach pushed us to do back in college to prepare for football season, learning how to come ten times in an hour was nothing. And the great thing is that part of me now looks at sex as a sport or a competition. It gets to bring out the athlete in me.

I like to see how many times I can come and how many times I can make my wife come. We make it a game to see how many different positions we can go through in 30-45 minutes. It's great. It really brings out the competitor in me and a part of me feels like this is how my body was naturally meant to operate. The way I've been doing it all these years, I was not using what my body's given me. It's like my body was built to process calculus but I was simply doing first-grade math all these years. Now I'm finally utilizing what my body's given me.

TNG™: "Have you tried telling your friends about this, and if so, what was their reaction?"

G: "It's funny, because when I tell guys about this, they just can't get it through their head. They think it's impossible for a guy to come without ejaculating. It just makes no sense to them. I guess because that's the way they were taught. I mean, if you just had a first grade math education and you sat down and tried to do calculus, it wouldn't make much sense to you either.

But now that I've learned to separate coming from actually ejaculating, it allows me to stay hard and continue making love like I never thought I could have, like I'm a 17-year-old kid again. Like I said, this isn't something that I go through every time when my wife and I make love. Sometimes we're both tired and just want a nice, short romantic lovemaking session. But oh man, when we're up for going all night, it's nice to know I now can."

Still in shock, we next spoke to Bob, who also happily relayed his new enjoyable sex life to us:

The Nice Guys™: "So Bob, what was your problem before you became multi-orgasmic?"

Bob: "Here was my main problem. I longed for those days when I was 17. I mean, being a 42-year-old guy, I just can't have sex like I used to back in the day, 25 years ago. For a while it got really depressing and actually was a key contributor to my wife and I getting divorced. In fact, I thought there was never going to be a solution. I mean, sure, I could use Viagra, but even with that, I just couldn't go and go morning and night like I could when I was 17 years old.

Especially now that I am partially retired, I have a lot of time off. With my current girlfriend, I really wanted to be able to wake up, have great sex in the morning, have sex in the afternoon, and have sex again at night. What else is there to live for? Unfortunately, before I was multi-orgasmic, if I had sex in the morning, that was it all day, sometimes even for two days. That's how long it took me to recover and be able to come again. Honestly, I didn't think I was asking too much of my body."

TNG™: "So what is your sex life like now?"

B: "Now my sex life is totally different. Now when I have sex, I go and go and go as long as I want to. Sometimes if I'm really horny or really turned on, I'll come for the first time within five minutes. Sometimes I'll make myself go 20 or 25 minutes before coming for the first time. This first orgasm is always the most powerful. Now I don't let myself come, but I still have an orgasm.

Whether it's five minutes or 25 minutes in, this one always feels the best. But the great thing is, since I'm not coming, I don't lose my hard-on. I can keep going and going and I found that if I do keep going, I have more tremors about every two to three minutes after that. Now the tremors never actually feel as good as the first orgasm, but they still feel pretty nice.

The great thing is my girlfriend operates in the same exact way. She too has a really powerful first orgasm and then after that, she continues to have tremors every few minutes. In fact, I've been told by my sex counselor that my sex patterns are very similar to many women's. If I'm coming like most women are, I'm happy with that because it's been my experience that women get to have much more pleasure during sex than we guys do, at least up until now."

TNG™: "So do you ever actually ejaculate?"

B: "Now the great part of it is that I never actually shoot my load. My girlfriend and I just keep going until the tremors are starting to die down and we no longer want to go anymore. My erection then naturally just dissipates. The great thing is since I don't actually come, I can go again in the afternoon and even at night. I can have three-a-days. I can go three times a day! What 42-year-old man, not on Viagra, can do this?"

TNG™: "As for the learning process, was it difficult?"

B: "Well, don't get me wrong. There were some weird things that happen when your body undergoes these changes. Sometimes my body would just come when I wasn't expecting it. Other times, I would have an orgasm and then I'd have a delayed come, like 10 seconds later, my body would start shooting out cum. Other times, I would have an orgasm and shoot a little bit of cum. Sometimes my penis would contract a little bit for a few seconds. I didn't know what was going on. Sometimes I would just totally lose my hard-on.

But oh man, once you master this, your orgasms without coming feel much better than they used to when you did come. Not only that but I understand my body better. I understand what's going on all the time and I really feel what's going on when I have an orgasm. I can feel my muscles contracting. I can feel my heart rate increase. I can feel my body explode without actually coming. It's incredible!"

TNG™: "Does it still feel as good, even though you don't ejaculate?"

B: "Absolutely! It feels incredible! Well, the first orgasm at least. The first time I come it feels better than any old orgasm I used to have. After that, the tremors don't feel as great, but hey – I never used to have them before! They're just a bonus! Overall, the entire experience is *way* better than my previous sex life. And, I'm not tired after sex. I can have sex three times a day. What could be a better discovery for a guy heading into his retirement years?!"

After interviewing these guys and hearing their stories, we at The Nice Guys' Institute™ were so intrigued at the possibility of guys having multiple orgasms, that we went online and ordered a bunch of books. We flipped through a bunch of them but ultimately these were our two favorites:

The Multi-Orgasmic Man: Sexual Secrets Every Man Should Know by Mantak Chia, Douglas Abrams
How to Make Love All Night (and Drive Your Woman Wild) by Barbara Keesling

Now we're all practicing trying to become multi-orgasmic guys. The steps involved are a little too intricate and require too much detail for us to go into here. Besides, we're not yet experts on the subject, so we wouldn't feel right presenting the information. But we highly encourage you to read these books, and we hope that you have great success with this, as Cameron, Gabe, and Bob have. We'll definitely have an update for you in the future. Please visit www.TheNiceGuysGuide.com to learn about our latest findings.

Visit the site often as we are constantly updating it with new content, including downloadable e-books and e-reports, audio tapes and CDs, and video cassettes and DVDs packed with our latest discoveries. We also maintain information on our web site about upcoming coaching sessions, course offerings, and speaking engagements. Additionally, we encourage readers to e-mail us, either through our web site, or at TheNiceGuys@TheNiceGuysGuide.com. Finally, please also come by and sign up for our free newsletter to receive the hottest tips to help nice guys like you make themselves more attractive to women WITHOUT turning into jerks!

Chapter 10 – The Nice Guys' Guide™ to the Movies

A reporter from the *New York Post* recently asked us for some advice on seeing a movie with a woman. She was writing an article on how a couple resolves which movie to see on a weekend in which a romantic comedy and an action flick are coming out. As soon as she asked, "How do you resolve this battle of the sexes?" we realized that our response belonged not only in the *New York Post* but in our forthcoming book as well since guys everywhere face this dilemma at some point.

In previous books in *The Nice Guys' Guide*™ Series, we have discussed the two criteria to use when planning a date and the tough choice whether to contact a woman via e-mail or phone. Now we at *The Nice Guys' Institute*™ will share what we've learned about planning a date to the movies.

The first question the journalist asked us was how to select a movie. We explained that if it's the first date, it's wise to see the movie that your date wants to see, even if it is a romantic comedy that you're not all that intrigued by. My friend Alexis put it best:

> "I like it when a guy I've just started dating goes with me to see a chick flick. Because, you know, the movie's about two people getting together, and if I'm just getting together with someone, then that's who I want to see it with. Besides, if he's willing to see the movie with me, I get to see the lighter, more compassionate side of him.
>
> I'll admit that I might be a little worried if he told me that he sits home watching *Legally Blonde* every night. But there's nothing wrong with a guy seeing a chick flick with me. In fact, I think it's kind of sweet."

Given Alexis' insight, it seems likely that you'll rack up points if you suggest seeing a romantic comedy. However, there's a right and a wrong way to do it. There's no need to lie and pretend that you love to watch romantic comedies. Note the difference between these responses to a woman mentioning a romantic comedy that she wants to see:

> "Yeah, I'd love to see that movie with you."
> "Yeah, I watch romantic comedies all the time."

Notice that the first one is the truth; the latter is an outright lie. As we've mentioned, lies tend to make for an unhealthy relationship. Use the first response, and you'll have a great date. Utter the second, and you may find yourself watching *Legally Blonde* on DVD every Friday night!

The second matter we discussed was the importance of compromise to a relationship. When you're dating someone, compromise is essential to keeping both parties happy. If you go with her to see a romantic comedy this week, then perhaps she'll go with you to see the latest action flick next week. By the same token, if she goes with you to see a movie that you really want to see, you should suggest that she gets to choose the next movie you see together.

Here's one final piece of advice: Do *not* split up once you get to the theater. We've actually seen guys go to the theater and see their movie alone, leaving their girlfriends or wives to watch a chick flick alone. If you weren't aware before, let us inform you now: A date is no longer a date when you and the person you are seeing are sitting in two different rooms for a couple of hours.

Sure this might not seem like a big deal to you because guys typically care more about the movie itself than who we see it with. If there's a movie that we really want to see, we usually don't care who we see it with and don't even mind seeing it alone. Women, on the other hand, bond through movies, and thus who they see a movie with is extremely important. In fact, women "save" movies for people. On multiple occasions, we've invited a female friend to see a movie, only to be rejected because she was saving that movie for her boyfriend or husband. We've learned not to be offended by this because now we're often the guy who women save movies for!

So keep in mind the importance of watching the movie together when you go to the movies with a woman. In fact, if she wants to watch a romantic comedy, be honored that she wants to see the movie with you and not with some other guy!

AFTERWORD

Becoming a Nice Guy™ is incredible! When you approach women by showing genuine, sincere interest in them, rather than bragging about yourself, women will really enjoy being around you. When you have patience, instead of being the aggressive male that so many guys are, women will be amazed and shocked. When you invite women to do fun things that you know interest them, they will gladly want to go out with you. When you focus your dates on having a fun time, and making great conversation, rather than trying to impress women with how much money you can spend on them, your dates will be intrigued that you're so much different from other guys they've dated. Women will *want* to date you, *want* to sleep with you, and *want* to enter into relationships with you. It will change your life, as it has changed ours.

The next step is up to you. Being a Nice Guy is extremely powerful, so don't waste any more time. Try it today – at a bar, at a party, in a bookstore, wherever – the possibilities are endless! Refer back to *The Nice Guys' Guide*™ Series when you have questions, or e-mail us at TheNiceGuys@TheNiceGuysGuide.com. Tell us your stories. Tell us all about the great girl you met by using the techniques in this book and how she *gave* you her contact info without you even asking. We'll put the best stories on our website!

We wish *you* as much success being a Nice Guy, as we have experienced ourselves.

Good luck,

The Nice Guy™ & The Nice Guys™

Glossary

Bothersome Environments – One of three types of environments in which to meet women (the other two are Naturally-Inviting Environments and Moderately-Inviting Environments). Bothersome environments are the toughest environments in which to meet women, because you are interrupting them from some other activity. Unfortunately, bothersome environments are also the most common places to meet women. These include: bars, bookstores, concerts, subways, buses, restaurants, coffee shops, grocery stores, festivals, parks, and walking down the street.

CCR – It is the premise of *Make Every Girl Want You*™. It is an acronym that stands for Compliments, Compassion, and Reassurance. By sincerely complimenting women, showing them compassion, and reassuring them that things will be ok in times of need, you make women feel good about themselves. This makes women want to be around you. When combined with a positive, confident attitude, women will *WANT* you.

Category 1 Guy – One of the three categories of guys who traditionally got women. Category 1 guys are really good-looking.

Category 2 Guy – One of the three categories of guys who traditionally got women. Category 2 guys are rich.

Category 3 Guy – One of the three categories of guys who traditionally got women. Category 3 guys are famous (including local celebrities).

Category 4 Guy – The new category of guys who get women: a Nice Guy.

Direct Vouch – A positive statement about you from a female friend of yours to a female friend of hers. An example is, "Jen, you have to meet my friend Dave!! He is really awesome!!" Receiving *direct vouches* is one of the best ways to befriend new women quickly. As you develop into a true Nice Guy, you will receive more and more of these.

Dudefest – You know what this is! It's when you end up at a party or event with mostly guys and few single women. True Nice Guys know how to handle this annoying situation properly.

Emotion Matching – This is the key to compassion. By matching a woman's mood, whether it is happy or sad, she feels connected to you emotionally.

Golden Rule of CCR – If you don't have anything CCR to say, don't say anything at all!

Indirect Vouch – This vouch occurs when you and the girl you've just met have a close mutual female friend. This girl that you've just met will be much more receptive toward you knowing that you are good friends with a friend of hers.

Man of CCR – This is what you become once you've read and implemented what we suggest in *Make Every Girl Want You*™. This man compliments women, shows compassion toward them, and reassures them. He projects a positive, confident attitude toward women. As a result, women love this type of guy. This, in turn, makes even more women want him. Women want a Man of CCR as much as one who is rich, famous, or really good-looking!

Moderately-Inviting Environments – One of three types of environments in which to meet women (the other two are Naturally-Inviting Environments and Bothersome Environments). Moderately-inviting environments are, as the name might suggest, moderately easy places to meet women. Some examples include: a co-ed sports team, a wine-tasting class, the local chapter of your alumni association, and a church or temple. When women are in these environments, their primary purpose often isn't to meet new people. They are usually, however, aware that they will meet new people through these groups and clubs, and thus are moderately inviting toward men who may approach them.

Naturally-Inviting Environments – One of three types of environments in which to meet women (the other two are Moderately-Inviting Environments and Bothersome Environments). Naturally-Inviting environments are the easiest environments in which to meet women, such as at a party where a mutual friend is likely to introduce you.

Relinquishing Short-Term Sexual Desire – Conveying an attitude toward women that you are interested in them as a person, *not* as a sex object.

Subconscious Vouch – This subtle vouch is extremely powerful. This vouch occurs when you bring a fun, attractive female friend to an event with you, and other women there see you with her. Subconsciously these other women think you get along well with all women. They will naturally desire you more because they see other fun, attractive women who also enjoy your company.

Third-Party Compliment – A compliment you say to one person regarding someone who is not present. It is the complete opposite of talking badly behind someone's back. It is such a great feeling the first time a female says, "You know, you never have a bad thing to say about anyone. I love the fact that you are always so positive. It's truly refreshing to be around someone who always sees the good in people."

Vouch – The positive response a female has toward you as a result of something positive she has seen or heard about you from other females. There are three types of vouches—the direct vouch, the indirect vouch, and the subconscious vouch.

Appendix A – Questions to Ask a Woman That You Have Just Met

Here are some topics for discussion as you're getting to know a girl. These will allow you to make great conversation, and provide you with ideas for things to invite her to. Do not *ever* ask these questions rapid-fire. These are simply meant to spark conversation, not to be asked sequentially. Inevitably, a question will send the two of you off on some random tangent, allowing you to learn exciting things about her that you never would have thought to ask. That is exactly the purpose of these questions. If you find yourself going through this list in order, then this girl probably doesn't want to talk to you right now. Go talk to someone else.

Background
- So are you from <this city>?
- Oh, where are you originally from?
- Do you like <city you're from>?

- Have you lived there your whole life?
- Where else have you lived?

Current City

- So why'd you come to <this city>?
- How long have you lived here?
- What part of town do you live in?
- What part of town do you normally go out in?
- How often do you go out? (Politely)

Career / Job

- So where do you work?
- Do you like it?
- How long have you worked there?
- Where did you work before that?

School

- So did you go to school around here?
- Where did you go to school?
- Why did you choose <school>?
- Did you like it?
- What did you major in?
- Why did you choose <major>?
- Did you like it?
- Have you thought about going back to school?
- To study what?
- Where have you thought about applying?

Friends

- So, do you have a lot of friends from school who live here in <city>?
- Where did most of your friends end up moving?

- (Try to lead into discussion of cities you've visited or where your friends live)

Family

- So does your family live in <city>?
- Do you visit them often?
- Do you have any siblings?
- Younger or older?
- Where do they live?
- Are you close to them?
  - (Discuss your own siblings, their ages, where they live, and how close you are)

Travel

- Ask if she's been to any cool nearby places, such as a nearby beach, ski resort, National Park, campground, city, tourist attraction, college, vineyard, or lake. Try to get a feel for what she enjoys doing and where she hasn't yet been but would love to go.

Sports

- So did you go to football/basketball games at <school>?
- Are you a sports fan?
- What sports do you follow (if any)?
- Do you play any sports?

Entertainment

- What's your favorite TV show?
- What TV shows do you watch regularly?
- Have you seen any good movies lately?

- What are your favorite types of movies?
- What is your all-time favorite movie?
- Are there any movies out now that you want to see? (Try to be subtle; don't imply too much)

Appendix B – Date Ideas

Here are some ideas for dates, or just fun things to do with a group of mixed-sex friends.

Nature

- Boating
- Fishing
- Canoeing
- Lake
- Hiking
- Camping
- Scenic drive
- Beach
- Skiing / snow boarding
- Tubing
- Caverns
- Jet ski
- Water ski
- Biking
- Picnic

- Roller-blading / Roller-skating
- Walk a girl's dog in a park
- Fly a kite in a park
- Paddle boating
- Barbecue at a friend's pool (or apartment complex's pool)
- Botanical Garden
- Park or other nice outdoor spot
- Walk around nearby college campus
- Apple picking

Culture

- Museum
- Aquarium
- Zoo
- Vineyard
- Play / musical
- Other cultural spots (check local guidebooks)

Amusement / Entertainment

- Theme park
- Movie theater
- Rent a movie
- Miniature golf
- Bowling
- Shoot pool
- Comedy club
- Ice skating
- Water park
- Concert
- Drive-in movie
- Karaoke
- Murder mystery dinner
- Watch horse racing
- Watch polo match

Play sports

- Volleyball
- Tennis (become doubles partners)
- Driving range
- Batting cage
- Racquetball

Sporting Events

- Pro, college, or minor league

Seasonal

- Outdoor concerts in the summertime
- Horse races in the spring/summer
- Halloween
  - Hayride
  - Pumpkin picking
- Christmas
  - Watch the Nutcracker
  - See Christmas lights

Food / Drinks

- Grab lunch during the week
- Sunday brunch
- Grab a drink after work
- Ice cream
- Sushi
- Pastry shop
- Coffee shop
- Grab dessert
- Cook for a girl (***Girls love this!)

- Cook with a girl, or ask her to show you how to make a recipe. (You should at least be minimally capable in the kitchen to request this)
- Order Chinese food or a pizza

Shopping

- Local mall
- Popular shopping district (may be out of town)

Appendix C – Recurring Event Ideas

Softball

Here are some guidelines for building a softball team:

- Join a local city or county league; it should be quite inexpensive.
- Make sure you enter a co-ed, non-competitive league. Do not make the mistake of entering a competitive league. This will scare off and annoy the girls.
- You may have a choice of season length; try to keep the season to about 2 months. Games will probably be weekly.
- Roster size is usually 20-25 people; 10 players usually play at once.
- Invite 7 or 8 guys to join the team; save the rest of the roster spots for girls. Try not to invite any highly competitive guys. This will really annoy the women.

- Go to the batting cage as a team or call a team practice before the season; this will be a good excuse to get all of the girls together.
- Send out a weekly e-mail the day of a game, reminding everyone of the game time, location, and directions. Ask people to respond if they will attend. Include your cell phone number in the e-mail; inevitably someone will get lost or forget the directions.
- You won't have a problem getting guys to attend; if you ever fall short, you can easily find a male friend to play for the day (guys love softball and guys love women—what guy wouldn't join in?)
- You will have problems getting girls to attend. You will probably need to call around each week just to convince 5 girls to show up.
- This used to frustrate us, until we started using it to our benefit. We would purposely try to fall a girl or two short each week so that we could invite a girl we'd recently met to play for the day.
- Do *not* take winning seriously. It is quite possible that you will be really bad. The girls don't mind losing. What girls do mind are highly competitive guys. Don't be that guy. Once again, try not to invite any highly competitive guys to play.
- Consider drinking during the games. This probably won't be permitted, since you'll be playing in a city/county park or on school grounds. Mix something up in a cooler and sneak it in. If anyone asks, just say it's juice.
- The best drink is something sweet with a lot of sugar. We recommend mixing 1-½ gallons of fruit punch with a handle of vodka and a 7-lb. bag of ice. Beer or non-sweet mixed drinks will dehydrate everyone.
- Don't forget to bring the equipment (bats and balls) to each game, or appoint someone to be responsible for it. If you're drinking, bring 25 paper or plastic cups each week.

- Appoint someone on the team to coach. Choose someone who knows softball well, but isn't highly competitive. This will relieve you of the responsibility of keeping track of who hasn't played yet, and listening to people (girls) whine about what position you've stuck them in.
- Have fun with it! It's a bit of work, but in the end it's a lot of fun and of great benefit to you!

Wine-tasting

Here are some guidelines for organizing wine tastings:

- Gather a small group of friends (maybe 10 people) who all know each other.
- Get together once a week or once every other week.
- Taste a new type of wine each week. (Some popular reds are Cabernet Sauvignon, Merlot, Shiraz, Pinot Noir, and Chianti; some popular whites are Chardonnay, Sauvignon Blanc, Pinot Grigio, and Riesling)
- Have a different person host it each week; rotate through the group so that everyone hosts once.
- Each week, have everyone bring a bottle of the chosen grape. It's actually better to state that there should be 1 bottle for every 2 people (any more than this is too much wine). Don't state 1 bottle per couple; this will dissuade single girls from attending.
- With the "1 bottle for every 2 people" rule in place, this makes it easy to call up a girl you've recently met and ask if she'd like to join you for the evening. Tell her you'll get the wine. If things go well, you can suggest that she get the wine next week.
- As people arrive, have the host put each bottle in a brown bag. Write a number on the outside of each bag. Give everyone a wine glass and have everyone rate each wine by number. At the end, remove the brown bags and let people see which wines they

liked best. Then let your friends drink from whichever bottle they please the rest of the evening.
- The host may wish to request that people bring their own wine glasses.
- It is a nice touch for the host to serve appetizers. Cheese and crackers are always popular with wine.
- Send out a weekly e-mail reminding everyone of the host, location, directions, grape, and time. Build enthusiasm by stating how much fun it will be!
- Run the wine-tasting events for 10-12 weeks, and then move on to another activity.
- Wine tasting is a lot of fun. The group size will probably grow each week.

Activity Night

A varying-activity night, in which you get together the same night every week but for a different activity, is also a lot of fun. Here are some good activities to try:

- Ice skating
- Night skiing
- Movie rental
- Bowling
- Potluck dinner
- Pool tournament
- Bar night
- Board/card game
- Miniature golf
- Wine and cheesecake night

Other Recurring Events

Here are some more ideas for recurring events. If you come up with any more, please e-mail us and let us know:

- Get everyone to take a weekly cooking class together
- Get everyone to take a weekly dancing class together (girls love this)
- Have a monthly potluck dinner; host every month or rotate hosts
- Movie night
- Have everyone gather one night a week to watch the popular TV shows
- Plan around actual events, such as a weekly concert series

Quick Order Form (NGG2)

Web Orders: www.TheNiceGuysGuide.com
E-mail Orders: sales@TheNiceGuysGuide.com
Fax Orders: see www.TheNiceGuysGuide.com
Telephone Orders: see www.TheNiceGuysGuide.com
Mail Orders: see www.TheNiceGuysGuide.com

Name: _____

Address: _____

City: _____ State: _____ Zip: _____

Telephone: _____

E-mail Address: _____

Shipping & Handling: $2.95/book for all orders in U.S. (total is $17.90/book in U.S., except in Virginia)

Sales tax: Please add 4.5% for products shipped to Virginia (total is $18.57/book in Virginia)

Quantity: _____   **Total: $**_____
I understand that I may return any products for a full refund—for any reason, no questions asked.

Payment: ____check   ____ credit card:
Payment must accompany orders. Allow 3 weeks for delivery.

____Visa   ____MasterCard

Card number: _____

Name on card: _____Exp. Date: _____

Signature: _____